THE
everyday
arthritis solution

food, movement, and lifestyle secrets to ease the pain and feel your best!

by **Richard Laliberte**

with Virginia Byers Kraus, MD, PhD, and Daniel S. Rooks, PhD

Reader's Digest

Published by the Reader's Digest Association, Inc.

Pleasantville, NY | Montreal

Project Staff

Editor: **Nancy Shuker**

Writer: **Richard Laliberte**

Consultants: **Virginia Byers Kraus, MD PhD**, and
Daniel S. Rooks, PhD

Recipe Editor: **Leslie Glover Pendleton, CCP**

Copy Editor: **Jeanette Gingold**

Design: **Michele Laseau**

Prepress Manager: **Douglas A. Croll**

Manufacturing Manager: **John Cassidy**

Production Coordinator: **Leslie Ann Caraballo**

Reader's Digest Health Publishing

Editor-in-Chief and Publishing Director:
Neil Wertheimer

Managing Editor: **Suzanne G. Beason**

Art Director: **Michele Laseau**

Marketing Director: **Dawn Nelson**

Vice President and General Manager:
Keira Krausz

Reader's Digest Association, Inc.

President, North America Global Editor-in-Chief:
Eric W. Schrier

Photographer: **Jill Wachter**

Photo Art Direction: **Marian Purcell-Solid Design**

Note to Readers

Photography Copyright © Jill Wachter

Additional stock photography supplied by Brand X, Corbis, Digitalvision, Dynamic Graphics, and Photodisc.

Library of Congress Cataloging-in-Publication Data

Laliberte, Richard.

The everyday arthritis solution : food, movement, and lifestyle secrets to ease the pain and feel your best / by Richard Laliberte with Virginia Byers Kraus and Daniel S. Rooks.

    p. cm.

Includes index.

  ISBN 0-7621-0476-7 (hbk.)

  1. Arthritis—Popular works. 2. Arthritis—Diet therapy—Popular works. 3. Arthritis—Exercise therapy—Popular works. I. Kraus, Virginia Byers. II. Rooks, Daniel S. III. Title.

  RC933.L29 2003

  616.7'22—dc22

             2003015113

Address any comments about *The Everyday Arthritis Solution* to:

The Reader's Digest Association, Inc.

Managing Editor, Home & Health Books

Reader's Digest Road

Pleasantville, NY 10570-7000

To order copies of *The Everyday Arthritis Solution*, call 1-800-846-2100

Visit our website at **rd.com**

Printed in the United States of America

1 3 5 7 9 10 8 6 4 2 (hardcover)

US 4411H/G

Introduction

You want to move freely every day. You want to have energy every day. You want to eat well every day. You want life to be filled with potential every day.

What's stopping you? We hope you didn't say "arthritis." But if you did, we are here to convince you otherwise. For as painful and debilitating as arthritis can be, there are effective solutions emerging for the condition that will give you far greater mobility and far less pain than you might expect.

Not long ago, when a doctor diagnosed a person with arthritis, the typical recommendation was painkillers, rest, and resignation. But research has proved this a most misguided prescription. Today we know that:

> movement and exercise are among the very best remedies for arthritis;

> certain foods are rich in nutrients that can help your suffering joints;

> certain supplements can significantly improve joint health and healing;

> a positive outlook and an active lifestyle will go a long way toward minimizing the impact of arthritis.

What's terrific about these findings is that you control each. You need a doctor to prescribe a medicine, but only you can decide to take a walk through the neighborhood, or to eat shrimp for dinner rather than steak—and yes, shrimp is an arthritis "superfood"!

The Everyday Arthritis Solution was written to bring you the freshest, most effective ways to manage your condition. While there are a lot of pages inside filled with exercise photos, don't be fooled into thinking this is merely a fitness book. Look closely and you'll discover hundreds of clever hints and tips for managing everyday life with arthritis—the best foods to eat, the right supplements to take, even the best meals to cook.

And then there are the exercises. Please don't be intimidated. We believe we have put together one of the most usable, comfortable, friendly set of movements possible for people with arthritis. Sample them like recipes in a cookbook, and then turn to Part IV to learn how to put them together into 5- to 15-minute routines for your particular needs, your particular abilities. Research is showing that there is nothing better you can do for arthritis than to strengthen joint muscles and to keep on moving. Here, for the first time, is the ultimate set of exercises for exactly your needs.

Indeed, we believe we have put together the most thorough guide to date for self-managing arthritis. The doctors and writers who worked on this book are the very best in their respective fields, and the results show. So take control of your condition. Give these exercises, tips, supplements, and recipes a try, and we promise you, *every* day will be a best day.

Neil Wertheimer
Editor-in-Chief
Reader's Digest Health Books

table of contents

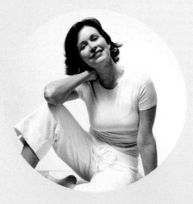

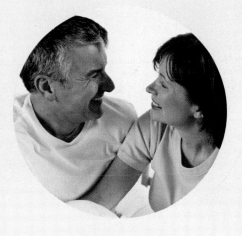

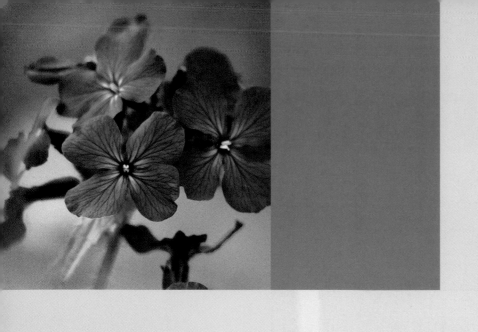

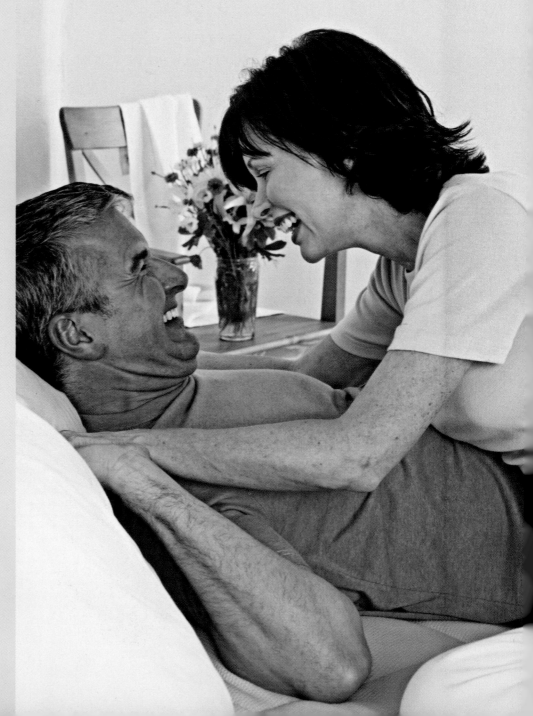

you can beat arthritis

When you have arthritis, it's easy to let scary words like

"degenerative" and "progressive" become stumbling blocks—

as if there's little you can do to ease pain and function better.

Nothing could be further from the truth. Arthritis may be

degenerative by nature, but there's plenty you can do to slow—

or even halt—its progression altogether. Exercise and a healthy

diet top the list of steps you can take, but they'll be even more

effective as part of a comprehensive self-care program that

uses all the comfort-keeping methods you can muster.

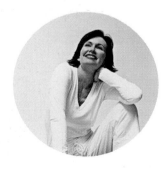

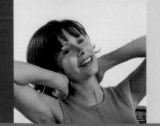
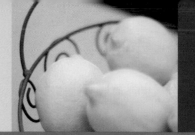

the arthritis action plan

A generation ago, the words "arthritis" and "action" were seldom spoken in the same sentence. Arthritis was considered a chronic, debilitating disease that inevitably slowed you down and ultimately left you hobbled. Action, on the other hand, was what arthritis prevented. Or so it was thought.

You live in a more enlightened time. Not that arthritis is less serious or pervasive than it ever was. It remains the number one cause of disability in the nation, and if you have it, you can take grim comfort in the fact that at least 43 million other sufferers share some form of your pain. No one has yet found a way to cure arthritis. But passively watching your function and mobility erode is no longer acceptable. In fact, action is not only possible with arthritis, it's the key to reducing pain and continuing to lead a productive, vigorous life.

Action against arthritis takes two forms. The first is fighting the disease itself with all the medical, physical, and psychological weapons at your disposal. The second is simply living life to the fullest—staying in action, moving your body, working your joints, and stretching your muscles. Living fully also means enjoying a robust and satisfying diet while controlling your weight and getting adequate amounts of nutrients that may help ease your symptoms. In short, taking action by living well promises to let you be even more active—and live even better.

Research pioneered at Stanford University shows that by using what scientists call arthritis self-management—in which exercise and healthy nutrition play a central role—you can tame arthritis pain, maintain function, and even make remarkable improvements. No more relying on doctors to tell you what to do. The self-management view puts you squarely in charge, enlisting doctors and other caregivers to support you with treatment and advice. Studies find that nonmedical habits, attitudes, and activities that you alone control often make the biggest difference in easing pain and enjoying life. Consider: Follow-up research has found that 20 months after learning more about exercise, diet, and other subjects in self-help courses (now widely available through local branches of the Arthritis Foundation), arthritis sufferers on average:

- reduced pain by 20 percent
- eased depression by 14 percent
- cut doctor visits by 35 percent

What's more, patients largely continued reaping these benefits as long as four years after first learning to call their own shots.

This book provides detailed information and advice on how to harness the power of exercise and good nutrition to beat back arthritis. But these elements fit into a bigger plan built on a variety of interrelated strategies. Other elements of a good action plan include:

Deconstruct your disease. Any manager needs information to make decisions, so the first step is to understand the basic causes, traits, and treatments of your condition. Just as important are the finer points of your arthritis. When does your pain flare? Which joints are affected most? How do you move your body to compensate? Answers to such questions determine what works for you—but not necessarily the next person. The more you and your doctor know about your personal case, the better you'll both be able to make smart choices.

Get a medical assist. Some of the most exciting recent advances in all of medicine have been new, potent drugs for controlling arthritis pain and the processes that cause it. Medications can establish a foundation of control over arthritis that makes it easier to build an exercise program and stick with it. With more options than ever before, ask your doctor for new recommendations if drugs you take have tough-to-tolerate side effects or aren't as effective as you'd like.

Control pain. Exercise can help you get rid of pain—but pain may also keep you from exercising. To make a breakout from pain, you may need to look beyond arthritis-specific or anti-inflammatory medications to effective mind-body therapies and, if necessary, more potent painkillers.

Focus on function. Relieving pain is the ultimate goal—or is it? Some would argue that you can't always use pain as the gauge for success. Instead, you should aim to restore, build, or maintain function. Even if moving your body causes some initial discomfort, making muscles stronger and increasing your range of motion can improve your quality of life and ultimately cut your pain.

Manage weight. For many people with osteoarthritis—the most common form of arthritis—carrying excess pounds puts added stress on damaged joints, making pain worse and accelerating the underlying deterioration. Losing weight with exercise and good nutrition causes a cascade of benefits in which you ease pain, gain mobility, and improve overall health.

Set objectives. None of these action items will happen on their own. And they won't happen at all unless you identify specific, realistic goals. Your goal may be to play tennis again or to dance at a child's wedding. Whatever your objectives, you'll need to decide on specific steps such as using this book to create an exercise program in order to meet them. Draw up detailed plans describing what you'll do and when, keep track of your progress, and continue setting new goals to keep moving ahead.

Adopt a can-do attitude. Are you determined to make a change? You should be. Not only will the steps you take pay positive dividends, just thinking positively can lead to improvements. Studies suggest that if you're confident you can control arthritis, you'll experience less pain and enjoy greater function than you would with a more pessimistic attitude. In some cases, the effects have been similar to those gained from nonsteroidal anti-inflammatory medications.

HOW TO HELP YOURSELF

The Arthritis Foundation offers a variety of self-help courses at local chapters across the country. To find a chapter near you, call the foundation at 800-283-7800 or log on to www.arthritis.org. Among the courses you can choose from:

Speaking of Pain
A workshop focusing specifically on pain—how to assess it, describe it, and work with health-care providers to relieve it.

Arthritis Basics for Change (ABC)
A self-management course that you take at home using audio recordings and related print materials.

Walk with Ease
Helps you develop a walking program that you can stick with to ease pain, manage your weight, and reduce stress.

The Arthritis Self-Help Course
Teaches skills in a group setting for building a lifestyle plan that's tailored to your needs. Trained volunteer leaders cover subjects including exercise, diet, pain management, fatigue, stress, and emotional obstacles.

People with Arthritis Can Exercise (PACE)
An exercise course that uses gentle exercises designed for people with arthritis to promote strength, flexibility, and range of motion.

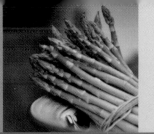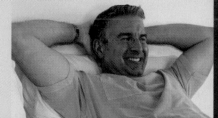

arthritis essentials

Arthritis isn't a single disease, but an umbrella term covering more than 120 different conditions. Self-care practices such as exercise and good nutrition can help control virtually any form of arthritis, but medical treatments, dietary goals, and exercise precautions can vary from one condition to the next. You don't have to know about every form of arthritis—just yours. And the vast majority of people with arthritis have one of two types.

Osteoarthritis: Crumbling Cartilage

When two hard bones come together in healthy joints, they're cushioned at their ends by a layer of smooth, slippery tissue called cartilage. Osteoarthritis (OA) gradually wears away this gristly layer, eventually exposing raw bones and allowing them to grate and grind against each other, which causes pain and swelling inside the joint. In some cases, fraying bone and cartilage set bits of matter free to float in the joint, prompting even more pain. As the body tries to heal the damage, especially early in the game, abnormal bone growths called spurs can form at the edges of a joint, typically giving fingers and toes a knobby appearance often associated with old age.

Osteoarthritis is generally considered a wear-and-tear disease that hobbles people as they get older, and most cases occur after midlife. But it's not entirely related to age. Younger people (about 16 percent of those between ages 18 and 44) can get osteoarthritis as well, especially women, who are slightly more at risk than men. You're also at higher risk if you're overweight, have a family history of osteoarthritis, suffered a joint injury at some point in your life, or have an occupation that repeatedly puts a lot of stress on specific joints.

While it's clear why osteoarthritis hurts, researchers still aren't sure why cartilage starts deteriorating. One prominent theory is that enzymes controlling natural breakdown and regeneration of cartilage get out of balance and cause progressive damage, but why this happens is a mystery.

Rheumatoid Arthritis: Attack from Within

If osteoarthritis is largely due to outside factors such as joint injury and genetic predisposition, rheumatoid arthritis (RA) appears to be an inside job. The basic problem is inflammation—a usually healthy process that occurs when the body's immune system is engaged in battle. In this case, however, the body's soldier cells mistakenly wage a friendly-fire war against good-guy cells inside your joints. The initial target is the synovium, a thin membrane that surrounds the joint. Under white blood cell attack, the synovium becomes painful and swollen. As the disease progresses, substances produced during inflammation begin eating away at cartilage, bone—and even surrounding muscles, ligaments, and tendons. Eventually, the entire joint may become unstable, weak, and unable to function normally.

Scientists don't yet understand what makes the body attack its own tissues—a category of illness known as autoimmune disease. But a number of factors are thought to play important roles. The fact that RA occurs three times more often in women—usually during the childbearing years—implicates female hormones. Genetics may help set the stage for an attack, but some environmental trigger may be necessary—perhaps an unknown virus or bacterium. Ultimately, RA probably involves a mix of factors, which may explain why it can vary so much from person to person. You may have a moderate case

ARTHRITIS at a glance

Although the two major forms of arthritis share the essential features of joint pain, stiffness, and swelling, they differ in a number of significant ways.

	Osteoarthritis	Rheumatoid Arthritis
Cause	Wearing away of protective cartilage, largely due to wear and tear or abuse, though genetics and inflammation also play roles.	Inflammation due to an attack on joints by the body's own immune system.
Age	Increasingly common with age, especially after midlife. By age 70, most people show signs of OA, though not everyone develops symptoms.	Overall numbers increase with age, but peak onset occurs young—between ages 20 and 45.
Gender bias	Before age 45, OA is more common in men. After 45, it's more common in women.	Three-quarters of all cases are in women.
Prevalence	By far the most common form of arthritis, affecting about 36 million people.	Though the second most prevalent arthritis type, RA is about 10 times less common than OA, affecting about 2 million people.
Symptoms	May affect only a limited number of joints—perhaps just one. Pain marked by swelling and stiffness is often most noticeable when you use the joint. Any joint is vulnerable, but trouble usually occurs in the fingers, knees, hips, and spine.	Can affect as many as 20 to 30 joints at once. Pain in a joint on one side of the body is usually matched on the other side as well. Flare-ups of pain marked by swelling and warmth (especially in the smaller joints of the hands and feet) may be accompanied by fatigue and general malaise. RA can also cause non-joint symptoms such as skin nodules and anemia.
Trends	As the baby boom generation ages, osteoarthritis is expected to affect 20 percent of the population by 2030.	For unknown reasons, research suggests new cases of RA may actually be dropping.

marked by flare-ups and periods of remission. Some people may experience symptoms for just a few months, while others may suffer persistently for years.

Other Diagnoses

If you think you have arthritis but don't have an official diagnosis, see a doctor to be sure what you're dealing with before launching into self-treatment. Early therapy appropriate for your condition has the greatest power to protect against further joint deterioration. Symptoms of joint disorders sometimes overlap and a bottom-line diagnosis may take time. But the sooner you nail it down, the better. Conditions your doctor may evaluate include:

Gout. Joint inflammation mostly in men caused by a buildup of uric acid, a waste product normally cleared by the kidneys. Gout is usually controllable with medication.

Lupus. An autoimmune disease like rheumatoid arthritis that, in addition to inflaming the joints, can cause body-wide symptoms such as fever, achiness, and skin rashes.

Low-back pain. Though most often caused by osteoarthritis, chronic torso trouble can also be due to muscle imbalances, disk problems, fractures, bony growths in the spine, and various diseases.

Lyme disease. A tick-borne infection, Lyme disease can usually be cured with antibiotics.

Ankylosing spondylitis. A form of inflammatory arthritis, mostly of the spine, this disease is treated with medication and flexibility exercises.

Research: What's Ahead

Newspapers seem to be filled these days with reports about arthritis. The reason is simple: Researchers are seeking solutions on many fronts, and progress is being made. Here are five noteworthy efforts:

1. Newly established standards for X rays that make images taken at different times more visually consistent will allow doctors to detect and track progression of osteoarthritis with far greater accuracy. Emerging use of MRIs will take arthritis imaging yet another step ahead.

2. By looking into the strange fact that osteoarthritis doesn't generally afflict ankles, researchers hope to understand the biochemistry of this protection and eventually identify drug targets that fight OA in other joints.

3. Geneticists are homing in on genes related to both osteo- and rheumatoid arthritis. Once genetic tests are in hand (they're already close with RA; an OA test may come by 2008), doctors will be able to prevent disability by screening and aggressively treating at-risk people earlier in their disease.

4. Recent research revealing that osteoarthritis has an inflammatory component like rheumatoid arthritis may someday lead to development of medicines on a par with those that have revolutionized RA treatment in recent years.

5. Harvard researchers say their discovery that an abnormal immune reaction to a type of carbohydrate in joints may be an important advance in understanding how RA develops—potentially a new avenue for finding novel treatments.

FIGHTING FIBROMYALGIA

Though not technically a form of arthritis, the painful condition known as fibromyalgia often accompanies arthritis and is actually twice as common as RA. Fibromyalgia is marked by persistent fatigue and muscular pain that typically concentrates in multiple tender points throughout the body. All these symptoms only make arthritis pain worse. But despite its miseries, fibromyalgia doesn't appear to cause any lasting physical damage or reflect any known underlying disease.

The causes of fibromyalgia are mysterious, though hormones, stress, infection, trauma, poor sleep, and abnormal neural chemistry may all play a role. Lack of disease targets doesn't rule out treatment, however. Certain medications—particularly acetaminophen (Tylenol) to relieve pain, tricyclic antidepressants (Elavil, Endep) to balance brain chemistry, and sedatives (Prozac) to promote sleep—ease symptoms in many people. But one of the most effective therapies, aerobic

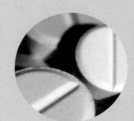

exercise, fits neatly into any existing arthritis self-management plan. Physical activity has been shown to ease muscle pain, boost energy, and promote better sleep in people with fibromyalgia.

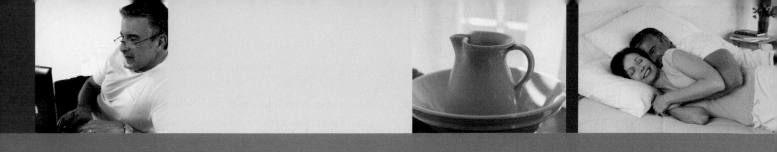

the medical arsenal

Even if exercise and good eating habits are mainstays of your treatment, you'll likely need extra control of pain and inflammation with medications your doctor can recommend. For both osteo- and rheumatoid arthritis, new drugs have transformed medical treatment just since the late 1990s. In the case of RA, medications are now able to zero in on highly specific pieces of the inflammation process and actually halt damage from the disease. There's still no cure, and after an initial splash, some drugs are causing ripples of concern about side effects. But your treatment options have never been better.

NSAIDs: The Old (and New) Standbys

Nonsteroidal anti-inflammatory drugs such as aspirin, ibuprofen, and naproxen may be the first medicines your doctor suggests, especially for osteoarthritis. They work by blocking the body's production of prostaglandins, chemicals that play a key role in causing the pain and swelling of inflammation. In addition to familiar over-the-counter brands such as Motrin, Advil, Nuprin, and Aleve, your doctor can draw from an extensive list of prescription variations, many of which are stronger per dose or are timed-release so they can be taken fewer times a day. A major drawback: Taken regularly, these NSAIDs tend to cause gastrointestinal problems such as stomach irritation and even bleeding. But a class of new NSAIDs known as COX-2 inhibitors (Celebrex, Vioxx, Bextra) now selectively suppress prostaglandins that cause inflammation while sparing others that protect the GI tract. Though COX-2s are expensive, their ability to relieve pain with far less stomach irritation has already allowed them to capture almost two-thirds of the arthritis drug market. They're not problem-free,

however: Side effects such as salt retention may make them poorer choices if you have heart problems.

The Weak NSAID

You'll find it on drugstore shelves next to ibuprofen and naproxen, but acetaminophen (Tylenol) isn't known as an anti-inflammatory drug. However, it is a good painkiller and, in moderate doses (up to 2 grams a day), can safely help arthritis patients to take lower doses of other NSAIDs to get relief. Taken in full doses, acetaminophen can irritate the stomach too.

DMARDs: Reining In RA

Disease-modifying anti-rheumatic drugs (DMARDs) live up to their name, actually altering the course of rheumatoid arthritis—perhaps even halting its progress—both by controlling inflammation and keeping joints from degenerating. Some DMARDs, such as the gold-standard methotrexate (Rheumatrex, Trexall), work by suppressing the immune system, but it's not entirely clear what makes all these drugs effective. The benefits are evident, however, and they're often used in combination, though it can take weeks or even months to see results. Most DMARDs were first used to treat other diseases such as cancer and malaria, but the recently approved leflunomide (Arava) was developed specifically for rheumatoid arthritis, part of a wave of new drugs targeted to RA. Side effects vary with each drug, but the powerful effects of many of these medications may raise risks of organ damage, especially in the liver. Some consumer groups have advocated a ban on Arava over such concerns, but other experts say that, while not right for everybody, these medications remain important options in the anti-arthritis arsenal.

BRMs: Hitting Tighter Targets

Like DMARDs, the new class of drugs known as biologic response modifiers (BRMs) can halt the progress of rheumatoid arthritis, but they work by targeting highly specific elements of the immune system. Etanercept (Enbrel) and infliximab (Remicade) block the action of tumor necrosis factor, a protein that triggers inflammation—as does adalimumab (Humira), which hit the market at the start of 2003. Another BRM, anakinra (Kineret) blocks a different protein called interleukin-1. All must be injected, though Enbrel, Humira, and Kineret are formulated so you can do this yourself at home. (Oral drugs are on the way.) Partly because they're inconvenient and extremely expensive—yearly costs can hit five figures—most doctors prescribe BRMs only if you don't respond to other drugs, but their joint-sparing effectiveness leads some physicians to recommend them earlier. While BRMs have roused a lot of excitement, their newness gives them a short side-effect track record. It's already known that some people taking these medicines may develop serious infections, and the FDA is looking into whether Enbrel, Remicade, and Humira raise the risk of lymphoma, a cancer of the immune system.

Corticosteroids: Blast from the Past

You might think stress hormones such as cortisol are all bad, but one of their natural functions is to help rein in the immune system. If you have rheumatoid arthritis, cortisol does this job less well, which is why corticosteroids—synthetic hormones—can help subdue inflammation and quell pain. Hailed as a breakthrough when introduced in the 1950s, they've since become notorious for side effects such as cataracts, gastric bleeding, facial swelling, and weight gain. But used carefully, steroids can be potent weapons. They're particularly effective in low (read: safer) oral doses if you have RA. And when injected directly into joints (up to three or four times a year without harming the joint), they can control inflammation for weeks or months without causing side effects throughout the body.

Managing Your Meds

To get the most from anti-arthritis medications, consider these pointers:

Don't hold back. Few people want to jump whole-hog into aggressive drug therapies, but studies suggest quickly hitting RA hard with medication and gradually backing off works better to spare you permanent joint damage than starting with less powerful drugs and working up to the stronger stuff.

Keep it simple. If your doctor recommends biologic response modifiers, ask about drugs such as Enbrel and Humira, which come packaged in pre-measured syringes.

Consider combinations. In some cases (Remicade and methotrexate, for example), two drugs taken together boost each other's effects.

Factor in total health. Sometimes your arthritis medication can do double duty on other diseases. Example: Taking an NSAID for arthritis can lower the risk of colon cancer or Alzheimer's disease.

Beware of interactions. Taking nonselective NSAIDs with low-dose aspirin prevents aspirin's ability to lower the risk of future heart attack. The COX-2 selective NSAIDs (Celebrex, Vioxx, and Bextra) do not interfere with aspirin's effectiveness.

Balance cost and effectiveness. New targeted drugs for RA are expensive, but studies suggest their ability to get people back to work and reduce other medical expenses makes them pay off in the long run.

Arthritis Drug Time Line

1898 Aspirin	**1949** Cortisone	**1974** Ibuprofen
1929 Gold salts	**1950** Acetaminophen	

A Shot of Relief for Knees

An injection of hyaluronic acid (Hylagen, Synvisc), a natural fluid found in healthy joints, can sometimes help stiff osteoarthritic knees loosen up and feel better after a series of three or five weekly injections. This jelly-like visco supplement may offer six months of pain relief.

Surgical Options

Joint operations are common for people who can't get rid of pain even at rest, have lost normal function, or haven't been helped by other treatments. Only you and your doctor can decide which operation might be appropriate for you. Options include correcting bone deformities (osteotomy); taking bone away from stiff joints so more pliable scar tissue can fill in the space (resection); pinning bones together so they're stiffer but better able to bear weight (fusion); removing the deteriorating synovium (synovectomy); and total joint replacement.

On the Treatment Horizon

Recent advances aside, even more treatment innovations may be in store in the near future.

1. It's already possible—but not yet practical—to take cartilage cells from your healthy joints, grow new ones in the lab, then inject these into an arthritic joint to shore it up. Scientists are fine-tuning the process of getting the new tissues to take hold.

2. Preliminary trials suggest that injecting joints with genes that suppress specific immune system functions may hold great promise for new treatments of rheumatoid arthritis.

3. Research continues on an old antibiotic called doxycycline, on a new mission. Early studies suggest it may prevent enzymes from breaking down cartilage.

4. Drugs called bisphosphonates (Fosamax, Actonel) that are used to treat osteoporosis have also been shown to slow cartilage breakdown in animals. Large trials in people are in progress.

WHO'S ON YOUR TEAM?

You may be managing your own care, but it's nice to know there's lots of help available when you need it. Whom should you turn to for what? The short list of specialists you may want to bring on board includes:

> **Rheumatologists**
Medical doctors who specialize in the treatment of arthritis and inflammatory diseases, particularly in the joints.

> **Orthopedic surgeons**
Medical doctors who treat bone and joint disorders and are qualified to perform arthroscopy, joint replacement, and other surgical procedures.

> **Physiatrists**
Rehabilitation doctors who treat chronic pain and physical disorders using physical methods such as heat, cold, electricity, and biomechanical adjustments.

> **Physical therapists**
Specialists trained to restore mobility and function using exercise and other physical agents, including heat, cold, and devices such as canes, braces, and special tools.

> **Occupational therapists**
Specialists who devise ways to make every day tasks such as cooking, driving, or getting dressed easier.

> **Chiropractors**
Health-care professionals who attempt to relieve pain and improve function by manipulating the spine and joints.

> **Acupuncturists**
Alternative practitioners who use fine needles to treat pain and other health problems.

1997 Visco supplements; disease-modifying anti-rheumatic drugs

1999 COX-2 inhibitors; biologic response modifiers

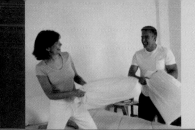
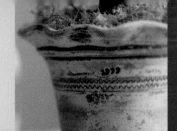
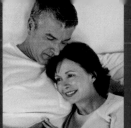

managing pain

Relieving pain has always been one of the chief goals of medicine, yet doctors traditionally haven't addressed it as a separate problem, focusing instead on underlying diseases. That perspective is changing as studies find that relieving pain helps people fight their illnesses better. It's now becoming common for doctors to view pain almost as a distinct disorder—or at the very least, a "fifth vital sign" (along with temperature, pulse, respiration, and blood pressure) that must be controlled for overall good health. Most treatments for arthritis both help ease pain and fight joint breakdown, but that's only the start of pain-control methods at your disposal.

Take Your Mind Away

It's clear that pain is as much a mental experience as a physical one. Ever get a sports injury that didn't really hurt until after you stopped playing, laughed off a bump on the head, or kissed away a child's boo-boo? That's the nebulous power of the mind at work against all-too-real pain. As pain signals zip back and forth between the brain and far reaches of the nervous system, they can be influenced in a number of different ways. One theory holds that gates in the nervous system's circuitry can be closed to pain if competing signals use the same pathway. That may allow you to curtail pain by filling your head with more pleasant thoughts through meditation, hypnosis, or exercises using imagery. Other research suggests that the way you interpret pain can change its impact on the body, making a sense of control, good spirits, and lack of anxiety potent buffers against suffering.

Picture Yourself in a Boat on a River

You don't need mind-blowing psychedelic excess to take your brain beyond your pain. You just need to focus on thoughts that are pleasant, calm, and engaging. Some of the best ways to do it:

Distract yourself. When pain flares, avoid dwelling on it by keeping yourself occupied. Any engaging activity such as reading, working a puzzle, watching TV, visiting friends, working on a craft, or going to an artistic performance can help. If you're stuck with nothing to do, try mind games such as counting backward from 100, listing the 50 states, or remembering the names of all your primary school teachers.

Meditate. Settle into a comfortable chair in a quiet corner. Close your eyes. Breathe deeply. Focus your mind on a simple word or phrase tied to your breathing. Those are the basic elements of meditation, which can ease pain by calming both your mind and body.

Take a mental trip. Wherever you go, there you are—but your mind can still be far away: strolling a beach at sunset, saluting the world from a mountaintop, or playing care-free in your old childhood home. To practice the technique known as imagery, picture yourself moving from one vivid setting to another. To engage as much of your brain as possible, focus on these elements:

● *Sensation.* Imagine how your whole body is affected by the soothing rock of a boat in calm waters or the wafting of a gentle breeze on your skin.
● *Smells.* Olfactory signals are closely linked with memories and emotions, and are thought to calm the same part of the brain that processes pain.
● *Colors.* Vivid hues are not only a feast for the mind's eye, they can also be used to represent your pain. Example: Visualize your pain as a red spot on your body that fades and dissipates as it's struck by the warming rays of the sun.

● *Temperature.* Imagined warmth is often more soothing (unless, perhaps, you live someplace oppressively hot). Imagine yourself in the temperate dawn of a tropical paradise.

● *Setting.* Picture yourself in locations you associate with relaxation or happiness—an island, a childhood vacation site, a favorite room.

Stifle Stress, Tame Pain

Stress is no fun for anybody, but if you have arthritis, it can actually be physically painful: When your mind is tense, it fouls your mood, which makes pain even more difficult to deal with. What's more, your body follows your mind's lead, and tense muscles translate to less mobility and greater physical discomfort. Exercise is a top stress-buster, and distraction, meditation, and imagery can help. So can the following:

Breathe deeply. Slow breathing that completely fills your lungs with air has been shown both to calm the mind and relax the body. To do it right, take your time (about four seconds) at every step—inhaling deeply, holding air in, and letting it out.

Scan your body. Tension isn't always obvious. In this technique, you systematically pay attention to the tightness you feel in every part of your body one area at a time, consciously allowing each part to relax as you breathe deeply.

Tighten and release. Stepping up from the body scan, you deliberately make each part of your body tight as your mind lands on it, clarifying the degree of tension it carries and allowing an even greater level of relaxation when you release.

Using Heat and Cold

Exercise isn't the only way to get physical with pain. The sensations of heat and cold can have remarkable pain-relieving effects. Cold not only numbs pain, it constricts blood vessels and helps reduce swelling. Heat enhances blood circulation and makes muscles relax. Both can help treat the pain of arthritis, though neither should be used for more than 15 or 20 minutes at a time. Some people find they get the best results by switching back and forth—treating joints with heat for several minutes, then (after resting a moment) following with a cold treatment for one minute.

When using cold. In lieu of refreezable commercial products, you can make your own cold pack by applying a bag of frozen vegetables or a sandwich bag filled with ice. It's best to wrap the pack in a towel to keep from damaging your skin. If you don't have a towel handy, keep ice moving in a circular pattern for several minutes at a time. Avoid using cold if you have poor circulation due to conditions such as diabetes.

When using heat. Heat comes either dry from lamps, heating pads, hot water bottles, and electric blankets, or wet from warm baths, steamy washcloths, or paraffin baths. Whatever you use, avoid combining these heat sources with a topical heating cream, which together can burn the skin. Don't apply pressure with heat, lie down on a heating pad, or fall asleep under a heat lamp.

TACKLE EVERYDAY TENSIONS

Sometimes it's the emotional baggage and little things that build up to big-time stress. To get a jump on them:

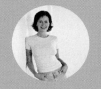

> Think, "I'm a winner." Failures and disappointments can make you waste time fretting over what could have been. First, there's nothing you can do about what's past. Second, you should challenge the concept of failure: Each setback was a step toward where you're going—and that's more important.

> Take a short view. Sure, the future may hold catastrophe—or not. Are you in a crisis right now? If not, don't sweat what may never come to pass.

> Embrace FAT—file, act, or toss. Keeping those your only options when handling paper will clobber clutter, a sure sign (and often a cause) of things feeling out of control.

> Spend face time with friends. Happy people tend to have real social networks. It's fine to chat with contacts on the Internet and follow the lives of oversexed sitcom friends on TV. But those people won't throw you a surprise party or meet you for coffee.

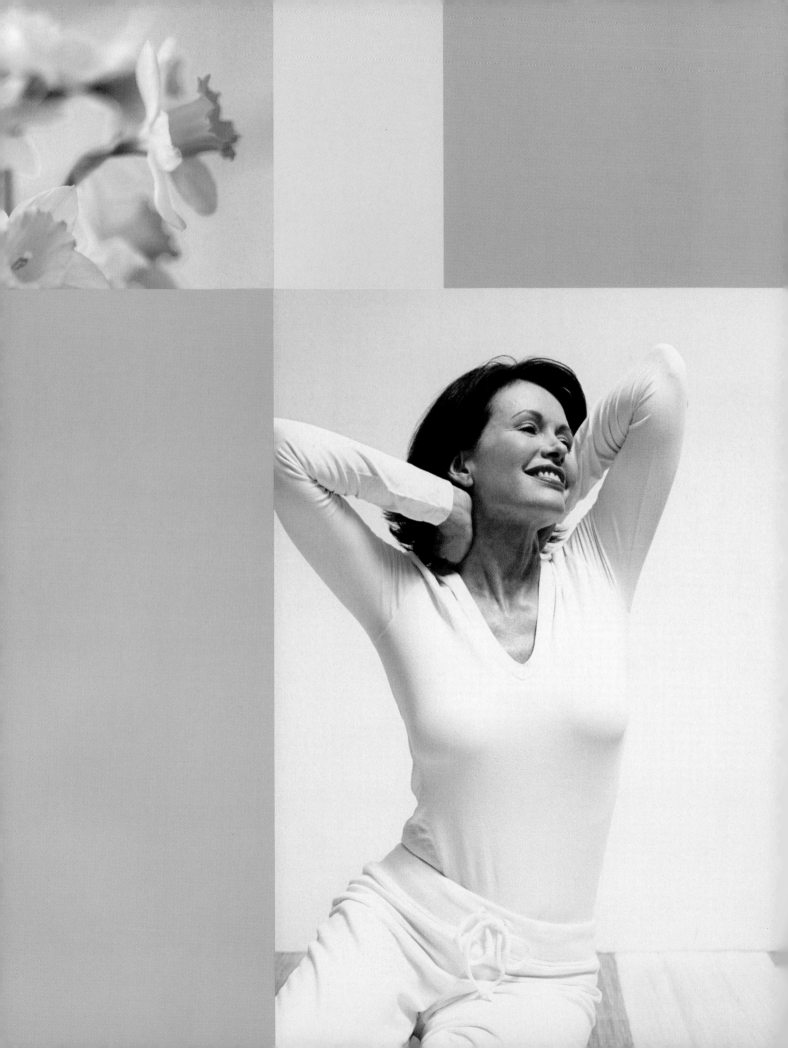

everyday
exercise solutions

One of the most powerful weapons against the crippling

of arthritis is neither a drug nor surgery. It is an old-fashioned

prescription for fitness: exercise. As a therapy for arthritis,

exercises are astonishingly effective, cheap, and safe.

If you regularly do stretches to keep limber, resistance training

to strengthen your muscles, and aerobic workouts for your

general health, you will improve your mobility and well-being.

No matter how much pain you're in or what your level of

dysfunction, exercises can make you better.

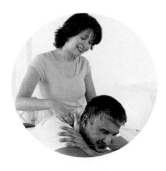

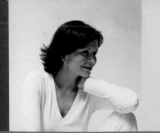

exercise as medicine

So much progress has been made in the drug battle against arthritis that some doctors (as many as half in some studies) don't tell their patients about the importance of exercise. Yet recent news about the curative powers of exercise for arthritis is just as exciting as research into new medications—maybe even more so. What drug costs virtually nothing, has no unhealthy side effects when used as directed, significantly improves symptoms of disability, boosts physical performance, and reduces pain? That's not just the promise of exercise—it's the documented result. Study after study has shown that you can ease the pain and constrictions of both osteoarthritis and rheumatoid arthritis with a wide variety of exercises. That means that no matter how disabled you may feel right now, there are exercises that can help you feel better.

Of course, exercise has its costs in time and effort, but both return handsome dividends. Motivating yourself to find the time and make the effort are challenges for virtually everyone who exercises. The greatest exercise challenge for people with arthritis, however, may be overcoming deep beliefs about their disease. Studies consistently indicate that people with arthritis, no matter what their age, tend to be less active than their healthy peers. And the irony is that the people with arthritis stand to gain even more from regular exercise.

What holds them back? Often, it is pain or the fear of it, fed by an age-old assumption that using your joints will make your arthritis worse. "It seems like a paradox," says Daniel Rooks, Ph.D., director of the Be Well! Tanger Center for Health Management at Harvard's Beth Israel Deaconess Medical Center in Boston. "If it hurts to move, most people move less.

But if you move appropriately to strengthen and loosen muscles, tendons, and ligaments, you can protect your joints, take pressure off them, and reduce your pain."

How can moving your body help ease painful joints, especially in the case of osteoarthritis, which is generally attributed to wear and tear? The answer lies with how joints are engineered. Shock-absorbing cartilage inside your joints is avascular—meaning it has no blood vessels to feed it nutrients and oxygen. Instead, the pliable-but-durable cartilage draws what it needs from surrounding fluid in the joint as it compresses and expands with use. As a result, using the joint makes cartilage more healthy, not less. (If using a joint causes pain, check with your doctor for the best approach to exercise.) At the same time, muscles support and protect joints, providing a strong buffer against stress and strain on cartilage. When muscles are weak and poorly developed, cartilage absorbs extra force, making it more prone to deteriorate, especially if injury or genetic susceptibility have already made your joints vulnerable to breakdown.

Exercise provides an antidote to these osteoarthritis problems by nourishing cartilage and bolstering it with construction of new muscle. With rheumatoid arthritis, exercise counteracts immune system overactivity that both makes joints deteriorate and robs protein from muscles, tearing them down and making joints more prone to further damage. And there's a bonus: Research suggests that exercising actually raises your threshold for pain. In one study at the University of Wisconsin, Madison, eight weeks of strength training in elderly people cut aches and pains associated with daily life by half.

How Your Effort Pays Off

Much of the most important research showing the value of exercise is relatively new. In fact, one of the largest, most definitive exercise studies, called the Fitness Arthritis and Seniors Trial (FAST), was only published in 1997. It found that when more than 400 over-60 people with arthritis broke into groups that walked, did strength training, or got a health education program, those that performed either form of exercise three times a week had up to 10 percent less pain and disability after 18 months than those who just got health lessons.

Some researchers, however, suspected that these widely hailed positive results were too tepid, and that significantly better outcomes were possible. Studies at Duke University have since found that doing more challenging (but not daunting) strength exercises using simple equipment at home can dramatically improve function and reduce pain by more than 40 percent. A more recent large study of more than 700 people at Tufts University similarly found that just 20 to 30 minutes of daily leg exercises using elastic bands significantly reduced knee pain and stiffness. The Tufts results were impressive, but only for the people in the exercise group who stuck with the program—about half the participants.

More Marvels of Movement

The ability of exercise to restore strength, shore up joints, relieve pressure, nourish cartilage, and expand range of motion would be more than enough to make it worth your investment in time and dedication. But when you have arthritis or related conditions, keeping your body moving has other benefits as well:

● It boosts energy and well-being. Keeping active helps control the depression and anxiety that often go along with chronic conditions, especially when they cause pain. It can also provide a sense of control, foster pride in accomplishment, and promote overall good health.

THE CHECK-IN CHECKUP

Consult with a doctor before starting any regular exercise program—especially if you have rheumatoid arthritis, which raises your risk of cardiovascular problems. You're not asking for permission to exercise. Instead, you're telling your doctor you want to become more active and need guidance on which activities are most appropriate for you. According to Virginia Kraus, M.D., Ph.D., medical director of the Arthritis Rehabilitation Program at the Duke University Center for Living, you and your doctor should factor in variables that include:

> **Your age**, overall fitness, and current level of activity

> **Your personal goals** and how well they fit into your existing lifestyle

> **Which joints are affected by arthritis**, whether they're in your upper or lower body (or both), and what patterns are evident—for example, whether pain occurs on one side of the body or both

> **How severe your arthritis is** and how it affects your daily life

> **Other conditions** you may be suffering from, such as fibromyalgia or osteoporosis

> **Surgeries** you may have had, especially in the joints

> **What has or hasn't been effective** in your prior treatment

> **How tired** you tend to be

> **Whether (and how much) you feel depressed**

> **Your eating habits**

> **Whether your footwear is adequate**

Adapted from *Textbook of Clinical Exercise Physiology*, Human Kinetics, 2003

- It helps you sleep. Chronic pain and sleep loss generally go hand in hand, and the resulting fatigue can make pain seem worse during waking hours. Compared to sedentary people, however, exercisers tend to fall asleep faster and wake up more refreshed even when they spend fewer hours in bed.
- It prevents osteoporosis. Although not directly connected to arthritis, many people (especially women) with osteoarthritis also have osteoporosis, a disease in which bones become thin and brittle. Exercises such as strength training can both help fight arthritis and add mass to dwindling bones.
- It fights fibromyalgia. Some cases of fibromyalgia seem related to sleep loss, so the ability of exercise to restore slumber can also ease symptoms of muscle pain. But beyond the bedtime benefit, aerobic and strength exercises seem to relieve muscle pain and tenderness in many folks with fibro.

WHY PEOPLE DON'T EXERCISE—and what to do

Arthritis can easily play a role in three of the top five causes of inactivity, as listed by the American College of Sports Medicine (ACSM). But, as the ACSM points out, none of these barriers need prevent you from being more active.

	Reason	Antidote
1	Avoiding discomfort from aches and pains.	Get tough—for now. Starting an exercise program is rarely easy and may feel uncomfortable at first, but you'll notice benefits quickly and discomfort will fade with time.
2	Modern conveniences such as cars and elevators take work away from us.	Work extra activity into your day by taking stairs or parking farther from your destination.
3	Leisure pursuits such as watching TV and surfing the Net are sedentary.	Find other ways to enjoy yourself—playing outside with a dog, for example, or creating that vegetable garden you've always wanted—that are more active.
4	Having a chronic illness makes exercise more difficult.	Acknowledge that exercise is crucial for fighting many diseases, including arthritis, heart disease, and diabetes.
5	An injury can make regular exercise uncomfortable.	Use targeted exercise for rehabilitation, continuing to work areas of the body that don't hurt.

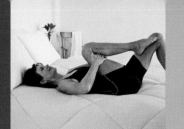
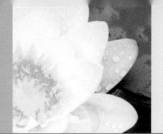
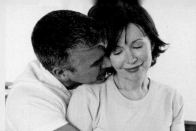

how to get started

Psychologists find that people typically move through several stages of motivation before taking any action. First, you become aware of a need for change. Next, you muse and ponder what to do. Then, you start taking positive steps to make it happen. If you've reached that point, you're already ahead of the game. You just need to forge ahead. Ultimately, your goal is to participate in a range of different exercises and activities, each of which has unique benefits to the body as a whole and to your joints in particular. These include:

- strength exercises to build joint-protecting muscle
- aerobic activities to increase muscle endurance, promote cardiovascular health, and burn calories for weight management
- stretches to improve range of motion and ease of movement

You'll profit most from a program that includes all of these elements—perhaps complemented by massage or movement therapies such as yoga. But don't worry if all the pieces aren't in place right off the bat. Regularly doing any single form of exercise will go a long way toward easing pain and restoring movement. It's wise, in fact, to avoid overdoing it in the earliest stages of an exercise program. On the other hand, drifting into a haphazard plan to "do something" isn't likely to achieve very good results. To make the most of a program, follow these guidelines:

Set specific goals. Goals imply commitment—which is exactly why you need them. But you should not be intimidated by goals. In fact, the whole point is to identify objectives that will be easy to meet, not hard. That way, you'll feel good about what you've accomplished and be motivated to make even more progress. Choose goals that are as specific and action-oriented as possible. Saying, "I'll do five stretches every morning" or "I'll walk through the neighborhood three times a week" is better than "I'll start being more active" or "I'll try to lose weight."

Start easy. Exercise won't cause more pain—if you do it correctly. Overdoing it, especially at the outset, can aggravate joint pain and cause normal muscle soreness, both of which will discourage you from sticking with your program. Talk to your doctor. If walking causes knee pain, for example, you may want to start by strengthening your thigh muscles, which will build support for the joints and make walking easier. Start with easy exercises to strengthen the quadriceps at the front of the thigh, and gradually work your way to more challenging resistance as you get stronger.

Keep records. You'll certainly notice differences in your strength and mobility over time, but for a shorter-term sense of progress and accomplishment, keep track of what you do—for example, how far (or long) you walk, how many times you can lift a weight, or how long you can hold a stretch. Write it down—and look back on how you've improved. Need help? Use your computer to log on free to an Internet fitness journal such as FitDay.com, where you can track and analyze both your daily exercise activities and eating habits.

Consider classes. You may find it easier to stay motivated in exercise classes tailored to people with arthritis. You'll benefit from getting expert instruction and you may find it more fun to interact with other exercisers.

But do what you like. If classroom exercise isn't your cup of tea, find a form of exercise you'll like better—swimming, biking, hiking. Your exercise may be a serious commitment, but that doesn't mean it can't be fun. In fact, many experts consider the choice of an exercise you enjoy—and likely will keep doing—to be the most critical exercise decision you make.

What If It Hurts?

Not all pain is bad—or to be avoided. You can expect to experience a certain amount of muscle soreness, especially if you're just starting a program after a long period of inactivity. Don't let it discourage you—it's actually a positive sign that you're challenging and strengthening your body. Starting out easy will help keep this post-workout soreness from making you too uncomfortable. Remember that discomfort from exercise usually dissipates quickly, and is less likely to recur the more you work out. A lot of discomfort may mean you are doing too much and should slow down.

Doctors make a distinction between achiness from exercise and pain that arises from arthritis. "The sensation from arthritis can be 'ouch!' pain," says Daniel Rooks, Ph.D., of Harvard's Beth Israel Deaconess Medical Center. "It's a much sharper pain that really feels like something is wrong, where pain from exercise is more of a soreness." How should you deal with the two types of pain? Here are some suggestions:

- Cushion the force on joints by doing low-impact activities such as walking, biking, or swimming.
- If muscle soreness lasts more than two days after exercising, you've probably overdone it. Next time, tone down the intensity of your workout by, for example, using lighter weights, doing fewer repetitions, or shortening your workout.
- If you feel sharp pain while exercising, stop what you're doing and don't start again until the pain goes away. Back off on the intensity until you can do the exercise without pain. If pain persists, see your doctor.
- Wear high-quality athletic footwear with ample cushioning and support to ease pressure on lower-body joints.
- If pain from rheumatoid arthritis flares, continue stretching and simple range-of-motion exercises in the unaffected joints until the flare-up dies down. Just make sure you get moving on the full program again as soon as you're able.
- If joints hurt or swell after exercising, apply ice for about 20 minutes following your workout and ease up on your next session.

WHERE TO TURN FOR HELP

Many hospitals offer arthritis rehabilitation programs, and the

Arthritis Foundation
(800-283-7800 or
www.arthritis.org)

provides both information and classes nationwide. But there are plenty of other places people with arthritis can find exercise instruction and/or classes. To find a program or get more information, try contacting:

The YMCA/YWCA
Both organizations feature exercise programs for older people, ranging from general fitness classes to pool-based water exercise courses. Call your local chapter for class offerings and schedules.

Community centers
Local health or senior centers often sponsor exercise classes appropriate for people with arthritis. Check the yellow pages under "senior citizen service" or "health-care centers" for local locations.

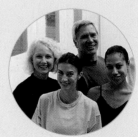

WILLPOWER FOR WORKING OUT

The exercises you start with aren't very hard. Sticking with them until the payoff is sometimes tough. Here are some ways to sustain your will to succeed:

> Underbook your bouts

It's vital to keep your goals realistic so you don't lose credibility with yourself. One way to do it: Commit to do less than you think you can. Sound defeatist? Look at it this way: It's better to promise yourself to exercise twice a week and hit both workouts than to say you'll exercise three times a week, then skip one session most weeks. Psychologically, you'll feel more satisfied and confident making all your dates. And if you actually do more than you committed yourself to, you'll feel particularly good about that.

> Exercise early if possible

To the extent that morning stiffness allows, try to work exercise into your day as early as you can. Early workouts are less likely to be disrupted by the day's events than those scheduled for later. Getting an active start to the day also leaves you feeling good from the get-go. That can foster a sense of well-being that helps you make other healthful decisions, such as what you'll eat for lunch.

> Focus on what's possible

Don't be daunted by long bouts of exercise. If you can't sustain 30 minutes of effort in the beginning or don't have that kind of time, break your workout into shorter intervals scattered throughout the day. Don't dwell on what can't be done, but take advantage of the time you have.

> Watch for "shoulds"

Willpower works when what you're doing is, in fact, what you want to do. If you find exercise to be an unpleasant obligation, you're probably doing it for the wrong reasons—for example, because someone else wants you to. Look instead for what you get from a workout to identify a benefit that will change "I should" to "I want."

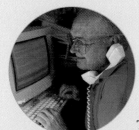

The American Association of Retired Persons
AARP's website, **www.aarp.org**, provides information on exercise for its members and the public.

Health clubs
The local gym may be full of muscle-bound people in spandex, but it's also a likely place to find classes appealing to people with more complex needs. Look in the yellow pages under "health clubs" or "gymnasiums."

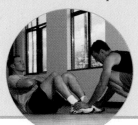

The American Orthopaedic Society for Sports Medicine
Check its website at **www.sportsmed.org** for a suggested 40-minute exercise program called TEAM—Twenty Exercises for Arthritis Management.

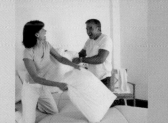
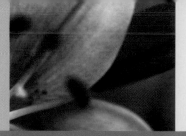

cardio: the whole-body workout

I t's been more than three decades since the term "aerobic" was lifted from high school biology (where it usually referred to bacteria that need air) and applied to a form of exercise that quickly morphed into dance classes and videos by curly-haired celebrities. But don't let the trendiness of the aerobics "movement" throw you. Aerobic (these days often referred to as "cardio") exercise isn't a fad—it's an element of human fitness as old as we are. In the past, people didn't think much about aerobics because they didn't have to. Working in the fields, walking where they needed to go, and chopping wood for the stove took care of aerobic needs automatically. Today, almost everyone could benefit from more aerobic exercise. And if you have arthritis, aerobic exercise offers above-average rewards.

Think of aerobics as whole-body exercise that has whole-body benefits. The idea is to engage in repetitive motion using large, oxygen-hungry groups of muscles such as the legs for extended periods of time. That boosts the body's intake of oxygen, which provides a workout to your heart and lungs. Working your cardiovascular system and muscles makes the body stronger and healthier overall, while the movement of exercise lubricates and nourishes joints, builds endurance, expands range of motion, and improves mobility.

You don't have to take special classes to participate in aerobics: Any activity that gets your heart pumping and makes you breathe more deeply will work. Some of the most natural forms of movement—especially walking—can provide aerobic benefits if you work your body intensely enough. Other forms of low-impact aerobics that are especially good for people with arthritis include swimming and biking.

Whatever form of exercise you choose, it's vital to work hard enough to get your heart rate up. As you become fitter, you'll be able to take on more strenuous challenges to maintain the same level of intensity. How hard is hard enough? Probably not as hard as you think. Studies find that you reap tremendous benefits from aerobics with only moderate effort—far less than is typical for conditioned athletes.

Getting into the Zone

To reap maximal aerobic benefits, you need to reach an ideal level of exertion that's neither too easy nor too hard. Surprisingly, most people tend to err on the side of difficulty, which can lead to injury. To get an idea how intensely you should exercise, ignore what anyone else is doing: A 20-minute walk might exhaust you but hardly faze the next person. But you can gauge how intensely you're working using a number of standards that work equally well for everyone no matter what your condition or which exercise you choose.

Method One: Hit Your Target Heart Rate

The classic intensity self-measure can sound complicated at first, but really isn't. If you can count the number of times your heart beats in 10 seconds, you've mastered the basic method. Here's how: Press lightly on an artery on the palm side of your wrist or on the neck to either side of your windpipe. Use a watch to mark the time while you count the beats in 10 seconds. Got the number? Now multiply by six to get beats per minute.

When you take your pulse this way while exercising, you get an idea how hard your heart is working. But this figure doesn't tell you anything unless you have one other bit of information: your target heart rate. This is the number of beats per minute you need to reach to achieve aerobic conditioning. Most exercise experts recommend hitting a heart rate that's 60 to 80 percent of your heart's maximum capability, which tends to be consistent from one person to the next, but changes with age. That makes it easy to calculate or (easier yet) plot in a chart like the one below.

Caution: The chart is for land-based exercise. Swimmers have different standards because the heart rate in water can be as much as 17 beats a minute slower than on land for the same work load. The Borg Scale (p.28) is a better indicator of intensity for swimmers.

If you're just starting an aerobic exercise program after being inactive for six months or more, begin at a low level of intensity. Some research suggests that low-level aerobics performed at only 40 percent of maximal heart rate is just as effective at conditioning the body, improving function, and reducing pain for people with osteoarthritis as more intense exercise at 70 percent of max. As you become more fit, you'll automatically have to start moving more vigorously to hit your target heart rate—and will be more capable of striving for an even higher target.

You can take the guesswork out of calculating and hitting your target heart rate by using a heart-rate monitor that does the math for you and may even chirp when you hit the rate you want. You can choose from an array of features (if you have poor eyesight, some even talk). But the basic function of all heart-rate monitors is straightforward. One part of the device picks up your heart rate either through a separate component strapped over your heart or one that's built into the wrist unit. The wrist device then dis-

HIT YOUR TARGET heart rate

Doctors recommend that you exercise at 60 to 80 percent of your maximum heart rate. Those just starting, however, might wish to target as low as 40 percent at first. Here are the targeted heart rates at various exertion levels, based on your age. To measure your heart rate, either use a monitor or take your pulse.

Age	Maximum Heart Rate (beats per minute)	40% of max	50% of max	60% of max	70% of max	80% of max
25	195	78	97	117	136	156
30	190	76	95	114	133	152
35	185	74	92	111	129	148
40	180	72	90	108	126	144
45	175	70	87	105	122	140
50	170	68	85	102	119	136
55	165	66	82	99	115	132
60	160	64	80	96	112	128
65	155	62	77	93	108	124
70	150	60	75	90	105	120
75	145	58	72	87	101	116
80	140	56	70	84	98	112

plays this information through a digital readout or an audible signal. Some units also tell you how many calories you're burning. Costs vary, but some units are priced less than $50.

Method Two: Trek with the Borg

Aiming for a target heart rate is the rational, hard-numbers approach, but there's also a more intuitive method in which you pay more attention to how exercise feels. A Swedish scientist named Gunnar Borg came up with a scale in the 1950s (now known as the Borg Scale) that measures what experts call perceived exertion. It has been widely adapted by doctors and researchers. Working from the chart below, inspired by Borg's model, you can gauge how intensely you're working out by the "How It Feels" criterion.

For aerobic conditioning, you'll generally need to work within the moderate or difficult levels of exertion. Avoid the very difficult level 5 to prevent overexertion. But don't feel as if exercise at the easy or mild levels has no value. Those are the levels of exertion you should aim for if:

- you're just starting an exercise program after six months or more of inactivity
- you experience a painful flare-up of rheumatoid arthritis, fibromyalgia, or lupus
- you feel significant pain from moving your body more vigorously

Method Three: The Talk Test

Perhaps the easiest way to gauge your exertion is simply to note how hard you're breathing. As a rule, if you're breathing deeply and working up a slight sweat but can still comfortably carry on a conversation without sucking air, you're probably within your target heart range.

Tweaking Your Intensity

Let's say you regularly hit your target heart rate by walking 30 minutes (an ideal amount of time for gaining aerobic benefits). But then something makes

THE BORG Scale

Intensity Level	Description	How It Feels
1	Very Easy	It hardly seems as if your muscles are working. You could keep up your activity for a long time without getting tired.
2	Mild	You can feel your muscles working, but you don't feel tired by the activity.
3	Moderate	You can feel your muscles working and still don't feel tired, but by the end of the activity, your muscles have to work noticeably harder than at the beginning.
4	Difficult	You can feel your muscles working from the beginning of the activity and your effort becomes noticeably harder about halfway through your workout. By the end, maintaining your pace takes a lot of effort, and you feel tired.
5	Very Difficult	Muscles work hard from the start and you're tired halfway through your workout. By the end, you're fatigued and couldn't repeat the activity without substantial rest.

COUNTING LONG AND SHORT

If you want to know your heartbeats per minute, does multiplying the beats you count in 10 seconds give you an accurate result? There's debate about the subject—and no perfect answer. How you count is up to you, but here are the pluses and minuses of different methods:

> **Counting for a full minute.** That's the number you're after, so why not keep it simple? This is, in fact, the most accurate method, especially if you count while you're exercising. Downside: If you count while resting, your heartbeat slows by the end of 60 seconds, skewing the accuracy of your workout heart rate. And if your mind wanders during the long count, you're sunk.

> **Counting for 10 seconds.** Beyond the fact that it saves you time, pausing for a 10-second reading multiplied by 6 provides a more accurate picture of how fast your heart beats while you're actually exercising. Downside: An error of only one heartbeat is magnified by a factor of six.

> **Counting for 20 seconds.** This is a compromise method that extends the count to protect against magnified errors, but is still short enough to provide a reasonably precise reading on your exercise pace. To do it, count as accurately as possible for 20 seconds, then multiply by 3 to get beats per minute.

a half-hour workout impossible—a change in your schedule, say, or a flare-up of pain. Maybe you could manage 10 minutes—but it hardly seems worth it. Have you been knocked off the exercise horse? Far from it. When there's a change in your exercise program, you can maintain the same level of overall exertion by making adjustments in one of three basic elements of aerobic training: how hard you push yourself, how long your workout lasts, and how often you exercise. Here's how:

● *If you can't exercise as long as you'd like.* Exercise more intensely in the time you have, or exercise more often in shorter bouts. One way is doing intervals: Push extra hard for 2 minutes, ease up for 2 minutes, then push for 2 minutes. Keep it

going until 10 minutes (or however much time you have) is up.

● *If you can't tolerate your usual intensity.* Exercise at a slower pace but for a longer period of time.

● *If you miss a workout.* Exercise longer the next time and, if it's comfortable to do so, strive for a slightly higher target heart rate.

● *If you want to crank it up a notch.* Add time, exercise more often, or work out more intensely—or make reasonable increases to all three.

● *If you're pushing too hard.* Back off on one or all of the three variables: how long, how often, or how hard you work out.

Aerobic Pointers for People with Arthritis

As a rule, try to avoid high-impact aerobic activities or exercises that put a lot of pressure on the legs, especially if you have arthritis pain in your knees or hips. Activities that are particularly tough on people with arthritis include jogging, jumping rope, and stair-stepping. On the other hand, some of the best aerobic exercises for healthy people are also best for people with arthritis. Even with these, however, people with arthritis should bear certain points in mind.

Walking. Walking is generally considered ideal because it's simple, low-impact, and requires little equipment beyond good shoes. As a rule, walking faster is a sign of improvement and a reasonable goal. But in some cases, walking faster puts added pressure on the knees, especially if you have poor biomechanics in your lower body. If walking hurts, check with your doctor: You may first need to strengthen specific muscles to ensure proper gait—or you may need to adjust your stride. For example, if you tend to limp due to arthritis pain, it's probably better for your joints if you take small steps with both legs rather than one short step and one long.

Swimming. The ability of water to provide resistance to muscles and take pressure off joints makes it a terrific

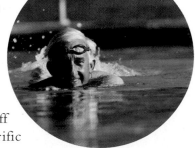

medium for conditioning if you have access to a pool. Avoid pool or tub temperatures above 98 degrees Fahrenheit, however, especially if you have RA: High temperatures raise cardiovascular risks. If arthritis in the neck makes it difficult to keep your head up for air while moving through the water, keep your neck straight by swimming with a mask and snorkel.

Bicycling. This is a great large-muscle workout that doesn't overly strain the knees. Outdoor riding is fun and freeing (though hills can put added pressure on knees), while indoor riding on stationary bikes allows you to watch TV, read, or listen to music while you exercise. Biking can be tough on the tush, however, especially if you have arthritis in your tailbone. The solution is a recumbent stationary bike, which is easier on the knees as well as the tailbone. If your hands have arthritis, be sure to keep a loose grip on the handlebars. Avoid straining against high gears at slower speeds: The pressure can put added stress on knees. And try raising the seat so that you touch the pedal with the ball of your foot rather than the flat bottom of your sole; the higher stance puts less pressure on the knees and hips.

FITNESS ON THE FLY

Exercise takes time. That's a given. People are short on time. That's a given too. But it's still possible to work aerobic activity into your day—either by carving time along the way, sneaking exercise into your normal daily routine, or boosting incentive to make your program a priority. Here are some ways to do it:

> **Broaden your definition.** Who says "exercise" has to mean "workout"? Fitness experts use the term "lifestyle exercise" to describe everyday activities that pay aerobic dividends. Examples include walking while shopping, doing yard work, and dancing.

> **Wear a pedometer.** Strapping on a device that counts your footfalls and clocks them in miles can be eye-opening—either because you walk a lot more than you thought or a lot less. Whatever the case, you'll have incentive either to build on your accomplishments or make up for lack of effort. In one recent study at Johns Hopkins University School of Nursing, people with osteoarthritis who received instructions on using a pedometer increased their daily walking significantly more than peers who received only arthritis self-management education.

> **Don't be auto-matic.** If you jump in the car for every neighborhood errand or visit to your friend down the street, pretend you've scrapped your wheels and use foot or pedal power for short-distance travel.

> **Use downtime.** Staring at the download bar on your computer screen doesn't burn any energy. But marching in place while you wait does. Anytime you're cooling your heels— waiting to meet a companion at the mall, for example— look for opportunities to take a short stroll, do toe raises, or perform some other physical movement.

> **Cut the chatter.** Social interaction can be an important way to keep exercise interesting and fun. But if the hobnobbing gets in the way of actually exercising or eats up time you need to spend on other things (which ultimately cuts workout time), break it off by, say, telling the other person you've got another commitment or suggesting you meet for a walk or bicycle ride in the park.

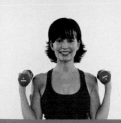
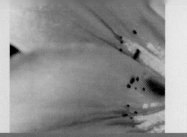
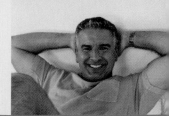

strength: maximizing muscle

If you want to be clear on the benefits of strength training for people with arthritis, take a look at what happens when you don't work to make muscles stronger. First, there's a natural decline in strength with age, just as there is with most measures of physical fitness. But that's minimal compared to the added declines in strength and function that pile up when you stop moving due to arthritis pain. In one 2002 study at Wake Forest University in Winston-Salem, North Carolina, people with chronic knee pain showed declines in knee and ankle strength as high as 7 percent, along with an overall loss of balance, over a period of 30 months.

But even if you've let your condition slide for years, you can restore your strength, regain function, and improve mobility far more dramatically than you lost them due to inactivity. In one recent two-year study in Finland, for example, people with rheumatoid arthritis who did strength training once or twice a week in addition to recreational activities made impressive strength gains of 19 to 59 percent! People who just stuck to recreation improved as well—but not nearly as much. What's more, the strength builders also made superior improvements in clinical measures of their disease, walking speed, and overall health.

Strength training differs from aerobic exercise in that it's performed over short, rather than extended, periods of time and aims to strengthen specific muscles or groups of muscles rather than the cardiovascular system or the body as a whole. If you're aerobically fit, you can walk to and from the supermarket. If your muscles are strong, you can carry a bag of groceries back with you. Strength, or resistance, training not only makes muscles stronger, it:

- boosts endurance
- increases tone
- makes muscles bigger
- adds thickness to joint-protecting connective tissues such as ligaments
- prevents bone loss and may even build bone.

When it comes to what kind of exercise you should do, it's not an either/or question: Aerobics and strength training have equally beneficial, but different, effects. It's best to do both. And in some cases (such as knee pain exacerbated by weak leg muscles) you may need to rehabilitate specific muscles with strength exercises before doing certain forms of aerobics.

Don't think for a minute that strength training is only for gym rats or professional bodybuilders. You're never too out of shape or too old to benefit from strength conditioning—which you can easily do with minimal equipment in your own home. Studies have found that even people in nursing homes can safely make striking gains. In one example, residents ages 72 to 98 more than doubled their strength in just 10 weeks of weight training, significantly improving their ability to walk and climb stairs.

Overcoming Resistance: What You Must Know

The essence of building strength is to work your muscles against some form of resistance such as a dumbbell, the tension in an elastic exercise band— or even the weight of your own body. How you start a strength-building program—and which exercises you choose—depends first of all on your level of function right now. If you can go about normal activities despite limited mobility or a certain degree

BONUS BENEFITS FROM BUILDING MUSCLE

Many people with arthritis suffer from—or are at risk for—other conditions as well. For example, if osteoarthritis is due in part to being overweight, you may be at risk for various forms of cardiovascular disease or diabetes. Though aerobics gets much of the credit for guarding against such conditions, strength training also has surprisingly broad benefits, such as:

> reducing blood pressure

> improving blood lipid profiles in people with high cholesterol

> helping the body use glucose more efficiently in people with diabetes

> allowing the body to burn more calories (and potentially lose more weight) by adding lean body mass, which requires more energy—even when you're at rest

> reducing risk of injury from participation in sports

of discomfort, the exercises you choose will be different from those you do if arthritis prevents you from performing basic tasks or keeps you in a wheelchair. But no matter what your functional level, you can improve your strength—and the exercises you'll find in this book provide a range of difficulty levels so you can make choices appropriate to your condition. Whatever exercises you decide on, however, the fundamental elements of strength training are the same:

Repetitions. If your idea of strength training is to spend hours doing complex programs or performing the same motions over and over (and then doing them some more), you'll be pleasantly surprised at how little time you need to spend on resistance exercises. As a rule, exercise physiologists find that you'll gain the most from strength training if you execute each movement only 8 to 12 times—as long as your muscles feel tired by the end

of the last repetition. If you're capable of doing more repetitions, the resistance is too light. (Doing a higher number of reps with less resistance is better for building endurance than strength.) If you're not capable of performing the exercise eight times, the resistance is too heavy and you're at greater risk of hurting yourself or making muscles too sore.

Tip: If you're using body weight as resistance (and therefore you can't lower the amount of resistance), do fewer than eight exercises if that feels more comfortable.

Sets. Strength-training enthusiasts will tell you that to get stronger, you need to do more than one set of repetitions. But there's debate about this. Multiple sets may make a difference for advanced bodybuilders, but studies suggest that one set of an exercise done at a challenging level is sufficient to bring about sizeable strength gains, with further sets providing minimal additional gain—perhaps as little as 3 percent. If you're motivated, doing a second set after resting a minute or two won't hurt—and you *will* progress faster. But doing a single set takes less time, may prevent you from overworking muscles, and allows you to concentrate your best effort where it counts.

Tip: If you want to add sets, wait until you've been exercising for three to four weeks. That way, you'll avoid taxing muscles too much at the start and give newly conditioned muscles a new challenge.

Speed. Working your muscles should not be a hasty business. To get the most out of an exercise, it's important to make your exertion steady, controlled, and *slooooww*. Besides reducing risk of injury, the slo-mo approach ensures that your muscles are working through their entire range of motion and that you're not letting momentum take effort away from you. The rule of thumb: Take slightly longer to lower the weight than to lift it. Some exercise experts advise a 6-second process—2 seconds up and 4 seconds down—while others suggest drawing each phase out by another second or so. But the most important thing is that exercises be both controlled and comfortable.

Tip: For an extra challenge that will draw out your lift slightly and help you maintain good control, hold for one second between the lifting and lowering phases.

Timing. How often should you strength train? Here, too, the answer may be less than you think. Researchers (such as those at Harvard, Stanford, and Duke universities) suggest you limit strength training to just twice a week—three times at most. It's important not to put muscles under continual strain, but to work them hard, then let them rest. Working your muscles actually causes microscopic damage to muscle fibers. When you allow muscles adequate time to recuperate, tissue builds back stronger than before. That makes *not* exercising just as important as the exercise itself. Just make sure you don't rest more than three days before exercising again—you'll quickly start losing whatever gains you've already made.

Tip: "Rest and recuperation" doesn't mean you can't exercise at all. Use your days off from resistance training to do light aerobic exercises—what physiologists call *active recovery*.

Getting into Gear

Most people can start exercising with little or no equipment—so don't let lack of gear hold you back. But as you get deeper into your program, especially for strength training, you'll need a few basic items—and maybe some extras to keep things interesting. Among the items you should consider:

● **Weights.** Though you can do many exercises using just your body weight, you'll eventually want to add resistance, and weights are a basic way to do it. There are a number of different types, and what you get depends on your needs, level of function, space, and available funds. Among your alternatives:

1. **Wearable weights.** Light weights that strap onto your ankles are handy ways to add resistance to leg exercises. Though you can buy them individually in a variety of weights, such as 1-, 3-, or 5-pound units, some products feature pockets that allow you to add or subtract weight (often in half- or quarter-pound increments) as your needs dictate. Given a choice between adjustable products that go up to 10 or 20 pounds, it's generally best to go for the higher weight. Reason: If you build up to a resistance greater than 10 pounds (which is entirely possible, even if you're just starting), you'll need to tap the heavier set for more resistance.

2. **Dumbbells.** These are weights attached to a short bar held in one hand. (If arthritis makes this difficult, you can also get strap-on wrist

TWO TYPES OF TRAINING

While the key to building strength is to work muscles against resistance, there are two basic ways to go about doing it. One makes joints move and the other doesn't. The basic breakdown:

Isotonic exercise. This form of strength training involves moving a joint through a range of motion against some form of resistance. The images of strength training that probably first spring to mind—lifting dumbbells or working on weightlifting machines—are examples of isotonic movement. Isotonic exercises are considered ideal for most people with arthritis because they closely correspond to motions you use in everyday activities, thereby efficiently helping to restore function.

Isometric exercise. With this form of exercise, you exert your muscles against resistance without moving your joint. In some cases, resistance is provided by an immovable object such as a wall. In other cases, resistance may come from weights or elastic bands that you hold in place rather than lift or stretch. While isometric exercises don't build strength through a full range of motion, they put less pressure on joints. That makes them especially useful for people whose joints are substantially damaged or prone to further inflammation from exercise. Isometrics are also useful for building endurance that you need for everyday tasks such as holding a bag of groceries.

weights.) You can buy dumbbells as precast solid pieces of metal, but a versatile alternative is to buy a bar (or two) with removable collars at either end, which allows you to put on and take off various-sized plates to adjust the weight. Use whatever feels most comfortable. If you buy an adjustable model, though, make sure the collars hold firmly and are easy to put on and take off. For example, if arthritis makes it difficult for you to squeeze spring-loaded self-locking collars (popular because they're quick), you might consider a collar that screws instead.

3. **Hand weights.** Hand weights consist of solid, single-piece cast metal shaped like dumbbells, but are coated with soft, colored plastic that makes them easier to handle, especially if arthritis affects joints in the hands. Hand weights usually come in light, easy-to-manage sizes, such as 1- and 2-pound units, which—along with their bright colors—make them look less "serious" than dumbbells. But you can perform the same types of movements with both kinds of weights.

● **Elastic bands or tubes.** Similar to oversized rubber bands, elastic bands or tubes provide resistance when they're stretched, but are lightweight and collapsible when they're not so you can carry them wherever you go. Different bands—often earmarked by varying colors—provide different levels of resistance based on the thickness of the stretchable material. Because pressure from stretched bands can be hard on hands, some products come equipped with handles or straps. You can do exercises to work every major muscle group with elastics, though it's more difficult to measure progress: While resistance from weights is measured exactly in pounds, resistance from bands is not easy to determine precisely.

● **A bench.** A bench isn't a must-have item if you're just starting a program—in most cases, you can get by using a sturdy chair. But when using free weights such as dumbbells, it's useful to have a steady platform to sit or lie on. A good bench can be inclined at different angles, and should be built for sturdiness: Look for heavy-duty tubing and a stable width that provides good shoulder and back support when lying down.

● **Fitness balls, sometimes called stability balls, physioballs, Swiss balls, or Resist-A-Balls.** Large, durable vinyl balls have been used for rehabilitation and high-level fitness training in the past, but have recently become hugely popular in the mass market. They're an excellent fitness tool because simple motions such as sitting or lying on a rolling surface forces you to make constant adjustments to maintain balance, which works a much wider variety of muscles than is the case with other forms of exercise. Balls are handy for both stretching and strength exercises,

STAYING ACTIVE—WHILE RESTING

By balancing strength training with aerobic exercise you can quickly and easily make physical activity a natural part of your daily life—with enough variety to keep things interesting. Here's an example of how you might balance the two basic exercise elements in a given week, while not undermining the effectiveness of either.

Monday:	Do resistance training.
Tuesday:	Let strength-trained muscles relax, but go for a leisurely bike ride.
Wednesday:	Take a class such as water aerobics, dance, yoga, or t'ai chi.
Thursday:	Do resistance training.
Friday:	Take a stroll with a loved one through the neighborhood or a park.
Saturday:	Do some light gardening or yard work such as raking.
Sunday:	Take a complete break—so you'll feel refreshed for the week ahead.

strength: maximizing muscle

and may add an element that's missing from many other types of exercise equipment: fun.

Running Your Resistance Regimen

All the elements are in place; now you need to start. Launching a strength-training program may seem daunting at first (especially if you have to buy yourself new equipment). But once you get going, there's nothing tricky about resistance exercise—as long as you take your time, concentrate on proper form, and follow your doctor's advice. As you conduct your program, here are some essential pointers to bear in mind:

Warm up first. Cold muscles and tendons tend to be stiffer, which limits range of motion while exercising and increases your risk of injury. Warming up by doing some form of light activity such as easy walking makes your body more pliable. It also enhances coordination by priming the nervous system for action and boosts the supply of nutrients to joints by increasing blood flow.

Breathe properly. You may be tempted to hold your breath while exerting your muscles, but it's important to breathe evenly throughout your exercises: Unless you keep oxygen flowing, rapid changes in blood pressure could make you black out. As a rule, breathe out slowly during the lift (positive) phase of your exercise, and breathe in slowly during the down (negative) phase.

Keep your body balanced. Make sure you exercise on both sides of your body to prevent muscle imbalances that could affect gait or function—potentially causing biomechanical problems that might make arthritis worse. For example, if you exercise the quadriceps at the front of your right thigh, you should perform the same exercise (with the same resistance, repetitions, and number of sets) on the left leg.

Rest between sets. If you do multiple sets, make sure you give your muscles a chance to recover briefly between bouts. The American College of Sports Medicine recommends a rest of about two minutes, but you don't have to be idle while you wait. Instead, do a set of exercises that work different muscles, then return to your second set—for example, alternate a set for the legs with a set for the arms or a pushing exercise for a pulling one.

IS STRENGTH TRAINING "UNLADYLIKE"?

Not by a long shot, according to the National Strength and Conditioning Association (NSCA), a professional organization. An NSCA position paper on the subject points out that:

> strength training has just as many benefits for women as men

> the same principles, programs, and exercises can be used by both sexes

> given an equal amount of lean body mass, women are just as strong as men

> in both women and men, resistance training can increase body muscle and reduce body fat

> because women's upper bodies are generally weaker than men's, women may want to work especially hard on upper-body exercises—traditionally seen as a man's domain

Progress gradually. As you get stronger, you'll be able to tackle more resistance—but don't make the mistake of piling on too much weight as soon as you start improving: You'll just end up sore or injured—and less likely to keep exercising. Instead, make incremental changes using the concept known as *progressive overload,* in which you slowly but steadily subject your body to greater challenges as it adapts. To do it:

● Start by adding repetitions. If you're doing 8 reps and feel you could do more, go to 9 or 10. When those become relatively easy, bump it to 11 or 12.

● Once you top out at 12 repetitions, add more resistance—but do fewer repetitions. For example, if you've been doing leg lifts just using your body weight, you might try using light ankle weights, but doing only 8 repetitions. From there, continue to add more repetitions as you're able.

● As one exercise continues to become easier, don't be afraid to start a different or more difficult exercise that works the muscle in a slightly different way—which not only keeps muscles developing, but keeps your workout interesting.

● Look back. If (as advised earlier) you keep track of your progress, be sure to look back after the first few months—that's when you're likely to see your biggest gains.

Quick and Easy Warmups

Warming up doesn't take a big commitment of time or effort. But a small amount of both will compound the impact of your strength training on joints and muscles. Some easy ways to prime your body for action:

- **Cardio quickies.** Do five minutes of light aerobic exercise such as low-impact walking or riding a stationary bike.
- **Light sets.** If you're already using weights or another form of resistance beyond body weight, you might also try very light sets of the same exercises you do to build strength. Just put your body through the motions with light resistance or none at all. Don't try to work to fatigue—you'll save that for the strength portion of the workout.

Pump Without Pain

Working against resistance raises the specter of potential injury, but strength exercises can be done safely if you keep the mechanics clean by using proper form. Some pointers that will keep you in tiptop shape:

- **Don't lock out.** Move your joints until they are almost straight. While exercising, avoid a locked-out position, which puts pressure on joints and increases the likelihood of further damage or irritation. What's more, locking joints such as the knees or elbows takes work away from your muscles and makes your exercise less effective.
- **Get a good grip.** If you're handling dumbbells or hand weights, be sure to grasp the bar by wrapping your thumb around one side and the rest of your fingers around the other for maximum stability. Avoid putting your thumb and fingers on one side, which will allow the bar to fall if it slips.
- **Place hands for balance.** When grasping a dumbbell or hand weight, grab it in the middle. If you can't hold the weight without it wobbling, it's probably too heavy.
- **Respond to pain.** If an exercise causes more pain, reduce the amount of resistance or do fewer repetitions—or both. Choose a different exercise if you're not comfortable, and see your doctor if pain persists.

Shortcuts to Strength

Some strength trainers are destined to become enthusiasts. But you may not be among them. If exercise seems grueling or dull, look for ways to make your hard-won efforts more effective and keep your workouts interesting. Here are some ways to start:

- **Gang up on muscles.** You'll see the biggest overall strength gains from what are called *compound exercises,* which hit large-muscle groups across more than one joint in major areas such as the thighs and chest rather than isolated muscles. For example, doing a push-up (or a modified version of one) will strengthen multiple chest, shoulder, and arm muscles, while a dumbbell fly isolates the chest's pectoral muscles.
- **Mix it up.** Eventually, any exercise reaches a plateau—a point of diminishing returns when continuing to do it no longer produces substantial gains. To keep challenging muscles (and stave off boredom), change your exercises or routine periodically. One simple change: Jazz up a cardio workout by breaking in with periodic strength exercises.
  Example: In many cities, pedestrian paths and parks are scattered with exercise stations that allow intervals of walking to be punctuated by simple exercises such as stomach crunches or step-ups.
- **Suck in your gut.** A hot topic in the fitness field these days is the value of building muscles at the body's core—the torso. Sophisticated training methods such as Pilates, which requires trainers and special equipment, have sprung up as a result, but the idea that a strong torso stabilizes the entire body isn't new. Nor are exercises to do it. One easy method: Make the most of your walks—even casual strolls through parking lots or malls—by toughening your torso while you amble. To do it, draw your abdominal muscles in as far as you can and hold for five seconds while breathing normally. Let your gut out and repeat. It's like doing crunches on the run.

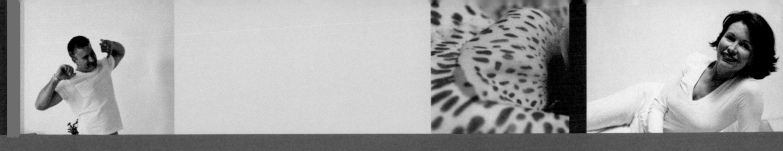

flexibility: graceful muscles

Challenging your muscles with aerobic or strength-training exercise is just one way to increase your mobility and reduce pain. Another is to systematically make your muscles more flexible through stretching and range-of-motion exercises. It's the difference between working your body and working *on* your body. The value of flexibility is easy to see: When muscle fibers become shortened through disuse or contraction to guard against pain, they can't easily move through their full range of motion—and neither can joints. In effect, stiff muscles hold joints back.

Lengthening muscles restores full range of motion both to muscles and joints, which improves mobility, boosts circulation to joints, and allows joint-protecting muscles to become stronger—all of which help ease pain. Stretching has other benefits as well. It's relaxing both for body and mind, making it a core element of body-movement disciplines such as yoga. Stretching also tends to make posture better and protects working muscles from becoming sore after exercise.

Flex Factors

When you think of improving flexibility, stretching is probably what comes to mind first. But it's also important to simply move muscles and joints through their range of motion. The differences between these two basic components of flexibility training:

Stretching. This is passive exercise in which you work muscles while they're relaxed. That's important because when you use muscles, they contract or become shorter—the opposite of what you're trying to achieve with stretching. Of course, your whole body isn't always relaxed when stretching: In most cases, contracting certain muscles is necessary to move in a way that lengthens others. As muscles lengthen, they become more supple, but (as with any exercise) you need to avoid pushing muscles too far, which can cause damage from tiny tears. Because warm muscles tend to be more pliable, stretches should be done at the *end* of a workout.

Range-of-motion exercises. Unlike stretches, range-of-motion (ROM) exercises are an active element of your routine in which muscles are put through their paces—but without straining them with extra resistance. The idea is simply to get muscles and joints moving in the ways for which they're designed, which works cartilage, boosts blood flow to joints, and primes muscles for further action. ROM exercises make good warmups for more intense exercises, so, although you can do them anytime, they're ideal activities for the *beginning* of a workout. If you're going to be swimming, for example, gently move your shoulders through the movements you'll use before getting in the water. Keep the movements small at first, then slowly extend the range of motion as you continue working your joints and muscles. Range-of-motion exercises are also an excellent way to overcome morning stiffness as you begin your day.

How to Do the Perfect Stretch

Stretching shouldn't be difficult, but to get the most benefit, you need to pay attention to proper form with each stretch. You'll find a variety of stretches for various joints described in the next section. No matter which stretch you choose, however, it's also important to keep a few fundamentals in mind:

Warm muscles first. Doing your exercise routine—or at least some light activity such as range-of-motion exercises—raises the temperature of muscles and other tissues surrounding joints, making them more pliable and allowing them to lengthen more readily with gentle stretches. Try to make stretching a follow-through routine every time you finish exercising, whether it's an aerobic outing or a bout of strength training. That way (assuming you're exercising as regularly as you should) you'll stretch almost every day—which is necessary to consolidate your gains, because elongated muscles tend to shorten again after a day or less.

Stay steady. Classic stretches most appropriate for people with arthritis are known as *static stretches,* and are performed the way they sound: Targeted muscles remain still while you lengthen them. Avoid stretching with vigorous motions such as throwing your elbows back to stretch the shoulders and chest—movements known as *dynamic stretches* that are far more likely to overextend muscles and cause damage. To do a static stretch, slowly stretch the muscle until you feel a gentle tug, which indicates you've

gone just a tad beyond the muscle's normal range of motion—a perfect stretch. Bouncing or pushing beyond this point won't help and is likely to hurt.

Hold at least 15 seconds. During the initial moments of a stretch, muscles actually work against being lengthened in a natural response known as the *stretch reflex.* Holding a stretch, however, allows muscles to relax and overcome their automatic tendency to contract. How long you should hold a stretch has been debated over the years, but most experts recommend between 15 to 30 seconds: Studies suggest that holding a stretch for a shorter period than this may be ineffective, while holding longer provides little additional benefit.

Breathe normally. As with weightlifting, some people tend to hold their breath while stretching, but it's important to breathe normally. In yoga, deep, rhythmic breathing is an integral part of stretching that adherents say contributes to the discipline's power of relaxation.

Aim for balance. Stretching helps promote good posture, but not unless you make sure your entire body enjoys its benefits. To prevent muscular imbalances, it's important to stretch muscles on both sides of the body, not just one, and to stretch opposing muscles such as hamstrings and quadriceps at the same session.

Quit if it hurts. Stretching should feel gentle, even relaxing. If a stretch causes discomfort, especially sharp pain, relieve the tension on the muscle or stop stretching. If you've had joint surgery, check with your doctor before stretching the joint that's been repaired.

The resting stretch. Don't want to take time after a workout to stretch? Try working stretches into the workout itself. One way to do it: If you perform multiple sets or rest between exercises in your strength workout, use the minute or two of respite between bouts to stretch. You can take it one muscle at a time, stretching the area you've just exercised, or do multiple stretches at once after your body is warmed up.

SHOULD YOU STRETCH BEFORE YOU EXERCISE?

For years, common wisdom held that stretching before a workout (after a short warmup) helped prevent injuries during exercise. But is it true?

At least two recent reviews of studies looking into the question concluded the answer is no.

One review author, an Australian doctor, had conducted a large study of his own involving more than 1,500 army recruits. All the soldiers were asked to do exercises such as jogging and sidestepping, but one group was allowed to do 20-minute stretches of the body's major muscle groups. Result: More than 300 subjects ended up injured during the 12-week study, but the mishap rate was about equal among stretchers and non-stretchers alike. While there didn't appear to be any harm in stretching, researchers conclude that it's probably more worthwhile to use pre-workout time for warm-ups and save stretching for your post-workout cool-down.

PUTTING IT TOGETHER: how to start

You've come to exercise, you've seen what to do, you're ready to conquer. But how to begin? Which exercises to choose? How much is too much? Just starting will make the answers come easier as you make adjustments through trial and error. But you can get a good idea of where your starting mark should be by evaluating your overall condition. If you've never exercised before or are starting after a long period of inactivity, here's how Daniel Rooks, Ph.D., director of Harvard's Beth Israel Deaconess Be Well! Tanger Center for Health Management, suggests you rate yourself and ease into your starting workout. Circle the number in the column that best describes how difficult it is for you to perform the following activities:

Activity	Very Difficult	Moderately Difficult	Not Difficult
Vigorous activities or sports such as lifting heavy objects, hiking, backpacking, soccer, singles tennis, or raquetball	1	2	3
Moderately intense activities or sports such as moving furniture, lifting and carrying groceries or a laundry basket, pushing a vacuum, scrubbing the shower, golf, bowling, or relaxed swimming	1	2	3
Rising from a chair without moving your arms	1	2	3
Climbing one flight of stairs	1	2	3
Climbing two or more flights of stairs	1	2	3
Walking for more than 10 minutes without resting	1	2	3
Walking for more than 20 minutes without resting	1	2	3

Scoring

Add all numbers you circled to get your total score. Use the total to find your function level below, along with conservative recommendations for starting points in the three basic elements of your fitness program.

7–12 points

Level 1: Low physical function
- Aerobics: 5 minutes a day, three to five days a week
- Strength: 1 set of 6 repetitions with an easy weight, two to three days a week.
- Flexibility: Hold stretches for 15 seconds

13–17 points

Level 2: Moderate physical function
- Aerobics: 10–12 minutes a day, three to five days a week
- Strength: 1 set of 6 to 8 repetitions with an easy weight, two to three days a week
- Flexibility: Hold stretches for 20 seconds

18–21 points

Level 3: Good physical function
- Aerobics: 20 minutes a day, three to five days a week
- Strength: 1 set of 8 repetitions with a moderate weight, two to three days a week
- Flexibility: Hold stretches for 30 seconds

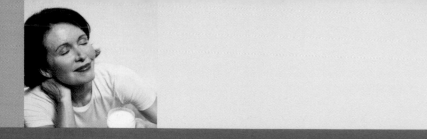
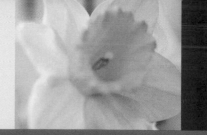

massage: beyond the pleasure principle

The feel-good power of massage to relieve discomfort, loosen muscles, and simply make you say "ahhhh…" is almost instinctive: Rubbing is likely the first action you take when pain or stiffness flares from arthritis or the minor dings and mishaps of daily life. Its seemingly obvious benefits once made massage a standard part of nurse education and a common treatment in hospitals. Advances in medical treatments such as drugs gradually pushed hands-on healing aside, but with alternative therapies gaining ground among both patients and doctors, massage is once again becoming a common way to help the body deal with arthritis.

"There's little data on the long-term benefit of massage for arthritis," says Harvard's Daniel Rooks, Ph.D. "But clinically, I can tell you that in some cases, it provides immediate benefits, even if those benefits may be short-lived." Among the claims made for massage are that it:

- soothes and relaxes muscles
- loosens stiff joints
- promotes greater mobility
- boosts blood circulation, enhancing delivery of nutrients to muscles and connective tissues
- triggers release of endorphins—pain-relieving chemicals produced in the body
- helps identify tender areas that may affect posture
- eases mental tension and anxiety, which can help relieve pain

Proponents of some massage disciplines go even further, suggesting that certain forms of healing touch or "bodywork" redirect the body's energy or teach the body new ways to move, improving overall health, preventing disease, and even helping you grapple with deep emotions.

Needless to say, not all of the claims for massage and bodywork are well supported scientifically. But it's worth asking why they need to be. If, for example, sufferers of chronic back pain say a month of twice-weekly massages makes them feel better when nothing else helps (as one study found), who can argue? "If it helps you relax, releases muscle tension, or relieves pain, that's the information that's important," says Rooks.

Bodywork at a Glance

Should you stick with feel-good Swedish massage or try one of a bewildering array of more specialized bodywork and posture-correcting techniques that may benefit people with arthritis? Only you can make that choice, but there's no need to read treatises on the theories behind each method. These are the basic differences that can help guide you.

Swedish Massage

Origin: Per Henrik Ling, a 19th-century Swedish gymnast, formulated the principles.

Theory: Relaxing strokes can relieve stress, improve muscle mobility, and enhance metabolic functions such as circulation.

Method: Four basic pleasurable strokes plus range-of-motion exercises.

Acupressure

Origin: Ancient part of traditional Chinese medicine.

Theory: Applying pressure at select points on the body (also used in acupuncture) promotes balance in "life energy," which promotes harmony and good health, and can relieve minor ailments.

Method: Pressure is applied to acupoints using the fingers and thumbs.

Shiatsu

Origin: Roots in traditional Chinese medicine, but developed in Japan in the early 20th century using modern understanding of anatomy.

Theory: Stimulating specific points harmonizes the body's energy. Energy patterns can be ascertained through a specialized diagnostic technique known as *hara*.

Method: Subtle finger pressure is used for diagnosis of energy through organs. Various touch techniques may be used, including stretching, squeezing, pressing, and rocking.

Reflexology

Origin: Built on ancient Chinese and Egyptian traditions but developed by various theorists over the centuries, most recently American therapists in the early 20th century.

Theory: The feet and toes contain "zones" that correspond to different organs and areas of the body. Stimulating reflex points on the feet can affect health elsewhere in the body.

Method: Foot massage using a variety of techniques, including "thumb walking," in which the thumb advances inchworm-style across the skin.

Alexander Technique

Origin: Frederick Matthias Alexander, a 19th-century Australian actor.

Theory: Correcting poor posture and bad movement habits can improve both physical and mental health.

Method: An instructor trains you to become aware of how your body moves, making corrections (such as keeping the spine straight) that can ease tension and pain.

Feldenkrais Method

Origin: Moshe Feldenkrais, a Russian-born atomic physicist and engineer.

Theory: Reprogramming habits in your posture and movements can correct disruptions in the nervous system that can lead to physical and psychiatric problems.

Method: An instructor teaches "awareness through movement" to correct poor movement and enhance function, while a gentle touch and manipulation technique known as functional integration helps improve mobility.

Rolfing

Origin: Ida Rolf, an American biochemist whose ideas first became popular in the 1960s and 1970s.

Theory: Loosening the fascia—a thin layer of connective tissue covering muscles—helps align the body with the forces of gravity and improves a wide variety of health measures.

Method: In a series of sessions, a practitioner uses hands, fingers, knuckles, and elbows to apply pressure—sometimes a lot of it—to tissue deep in the body.

Hellerwork

Origin: Joseph Heller, an aerospace engineer who studied with Ida Rolf.

Theory: Rolfing bodywork is not enough: You also need to explore emotions triggered by the release of tension.

Method: The deep-tissue bodywork of Rolfing is combined with movement re-education and a guided dialogue with the practitioner about feelings released by the therapy.

Tragerwork

Origin: Milton Trager, an American doctor and devotee of transcendental meditation.

Theory: Using touch to induce profound relaxation releases deeply rooted tension built through years of experiences and trauma.

Method: A variety of light and gentle touch techniques, including rocking, jiggling, and stretching, are used to create a feeling of lightness or floating.

Reiki

Origin: Mikao Usui, a Japanese theologian, from roots in Buddhism.

Theory: Channeling life energy at the atomic level promotes harmony and resists disease.

Method: A form of spiritual healing, reiki sessions usually involve a practitioner holding his hands on or near 12 different areas of the body.

Finding Good Hands

Your doctor can probably recommend a good massage therapist—and in some community health centers, the practitioner may have an office just down the hall. There's no need to scour dubious-looking storefront establishments or wonder what the "total relaxation experience" promised in a yellow page ad really means. Reputable massage therapists should be certified and meet professional standards established by any number of oversight organizations. Ask for credentials when you call for information or appointments, or check with one of these professional groups for referral to a therapist in your area:

American Massage Therapy Association
820 Davis Street, Suite 100
Evanston, IL 60201-4444

FOUR BASIC body soothers

Though there are many massage techniques, Swedish massage is the type you're probably most familiar with, and you've likely used its methods intuitively before. Unlike some bodywork disciplines, you don't need a specially trained or certified practitioner to benefit from Swedish massage (though enjoying the ministrations of a trained Swedish masseuse may certainly feel nicer) and many therapists recommend doing self-massage using basic Swedish massage techniques to sustain the benefits of a massage by someone else. Here are the essential methods and how best to use them:

Technique	Basic Method	Nature of Action	Self-Performance Pointers
Effleurage	Stroking	Long, gliding strokes using the whole hand or the pads of the thumbs. Strokes are often done toward the heart to promote flow through the circulatory and lymphatic systems	Move your hand over the length of a muscle in slow, rhythmic movements. In areas you can reach with both hands, keep both hands moving over muscles, following one stroke immediately with another.
Pétrissage	Kneading	Rhythmic compression and relaxing of muscles in a rolling, squeezing or pressing action	Without pinching the flesh, massage it deeply between fingers and thumb or fingers and palm. Work in rhythmic fashion, moving from one area to the next after 10 to 20 seconds.
Frottage	Friction	Deep, penetrating rubbing over a small area, pressing with the thumbs or fingers	Work in circular movements beginning with light pressure, but slowly applying greater (but not too much) force. To massage large muscle areas such as the thighs, you can also use the heel of your hand.
Tapotement	Drumming	A brisk, percussive action usingboth hands to tap or hack the skin	Use the sides of the hands to concentrate drumming energy. Keep hands relaxed and loose as you work, using sharp, alternating taps.

Phone: 847-864-0123
Fax: 847-864-1178
Website: www.amtamassage.org

**National Certification Board for
Therapeutic Massage and Bodywork**
8201 Greensboro Drive, Suite 300
McLean, VA 22102
Phone: 800-296-0664
Fax: 703-610-9005
Website: www.ncbtmb.com

Tools of the Trade

There's just one limit to self-massage: It's not easy to reach every part of your body that's crying for a soothing touch. The best solution: Find a willing partner. The second-best solution: Reach for a tool that gives you access to the inaccessible or helps make self-massage easier. You'll find a wide variety of options with a simple Internet search under "massage tools." Here are a few good bets:

Curved canes. With a variety of names such as Backnobber, Body Back Buddy, and Thera Cane, these curved and knobbed tools can reach over your shoulder and around your back to stimulate out-of-sight regions to your rear. You can use them to apply pressure even with minimal amounts of mobility or strength.

Jacknobber. With a shape like the objects you scoop up in a game of jacks, this tool provides multiple knobs that you can use to massage your body using different angles and multiple points of pressure. Placing it in a chair or against a wall, you can use it to reach points in your back, while placing it on the floor lets you apply pressure to the bottoms of your feet.

Bongers. Looking like a cross between something you'd play in a rhythm band and a kitchen utensil, these rubber balls at the end of a flexible metal shaft and a wooden handle can be used for both percussive and pressure massage. Because of their length, they can also reach areas behind your shoulders and back.

A CAUTION ON MASSAGE

Avoid massaging joints and muscles when you're going through a flare-up of pain or swelling from arthritis.

"During active inflammation, manipulation of the joints with massage may actually make your condition worse,"
says Bambi Mathay, a licensed massage therapist at the Harvard-affiliated Dana Farber Cancer Institute, and North Shore Heart and Wellness Center at Salem Hospital in Salem, Massachusetts. For this reason, some therapists suggest that only trained practitioners should do massage on people with arthritis, but others are not so rigid. Once a flare-up subsides, Mathay says, "self-massage is an easy and safe way to reduce pain and improve the health of joints."

Index Knobber. If arthritis in your hands makes it difficult to apply massage pressure or grasp other kinds of tools, the thick shaft of this tool acts as a mechanical extension of your hand, allowing you to apply pressure without overly straining joints in your fingers.

Foot roller. These come in a variety of shapes and sizes, some with knobs and others with ridges. Any of them allow a rolling action to apply moving pressure to the bottoms of your feet.

Tennis ball. For a low-cost alternative, use a simple tennis ball placed against a wall or on a chair to massage muscles in your back as you lean back and roll the ball with your body. To allow you to place it more easily, try putting the ball inside an old sock.

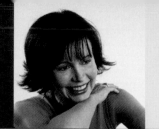
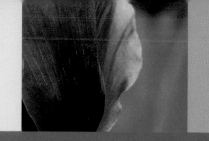

water workouts: wet, not wild

What if you could find a form of exercise that boosts the power of your strength workout, improves aerobic fitness, soothes pain, relaxes the body, and is exceptionally easy on joints? That's the promise of exercising in the water—which means more than just swimming. Swimming is an excellent aerobic exercise that builds muscular endurance, but there's no doubt it takes a certain amount of skill. That needn't leave you high and dry when it comes to water's fitness benefits, however. Even if you can't swim, exercising in the water is easy for almost everybody, and is good for you in ways that swimming alone can't beat.

Many doctors and physical therapists consider water exercise (sometimes called aquatics) the exercise of choice for people with arthritis. First, the buoyancy of water neutralizes about 90 percent of your body weight, taking stress off your knees, hips, feet, and back. Movement that is slow, controlled, and graceful is inherently easy on joints. At the same time, because water is 12 times denser than air, it provides resistance to your every movement, which builds strength by making muscles work harder in all directions. Think of a pool as the world's most sophisticated total-body workout machine—but more fun. Some of its finer points:

- Because water resists movement in all directions, muscles do double duty under the waves. In some cases, a single exercise such as running can work two groups of muscles (for example, the quadriceps at the front of the leg and the hamstrings at the back), while the same exercise on land would favor only one.
- You can quickly and easily adjust resistance almost without thinking about it simply by extending arms or legs or pulling them closer to the body (which changes your leverage), cupping hands so they catch more resistance as you move, or moving your body faster or slower through the water. A variety of tools, such as paddles or special water gloves, can help you add resistance.
- Even though water works your muscles when you move, the sensation of floating and the massage-like pressure of water also help muscles relax, which makes range-of-motion exercises and stretches easier and more pleasant.
- Water provides a boost to cardiovascular fitness because pressure from the water helps blood flow back to the heart and makes the lungs work slightly harder. At the same time, water exercise can seem less tiring because you don't get hot and sweaty.
- Because gravity stabilizes you less in the water, you make greater use of core muscles such as the abdomen and back to keep you steady and upright, which promotes strength, coordination, and balance.

Working in Water

Water workouts are simple and easy, low on pain, high on relaxation—and, for many people, just plain enjoyable. Beyond its physical properties and benefits, enthusiasts say water promotes feelings of well-being simply because it feels good, reduces stress, and washes away negative emotions. Still, you'll get the most pleasure and benefit from water exercise if you keep a few pointers in mind:

Practice basic precautions. Everyone understands that water also poses inherent dangers, but it's a sad fact that the dangers tend to take people by surprise when they actually cause harm. You don't have to dwell on this constantly: Just make sure you work out in a pool where qualified lifeguards are always on hand. If you have a private pool, don't work out alone.

Tend to temperature. The Arthritis Foundation recommends exercising in water that's about 84 degrees Fahrenheit. One concern is protection of people with Raynaud's phenomenon, a condition associated with autoimmune diseases in which cold can cause blood vessels of the hands and feet to go into spasm. If you're not sensitive to cold, you can probably deal with water temperatures a few degrees cooler, typical of many pools. To avoid getting chilly (and get the most from your workout), keep your body moving while you're in the water. Wearing a Lycra bodysuit with long arms and/or long legs can keep a swimmer warmer. You can buy Lycra bodysuits at dance stores or on the Internet from stores that carry active sportswear.

Watch entry and exit. Enter the pool using the easiest, gentlest approach. If the pool has stairs built into the shallow end, use those. If not, find the pool's shallowest depth, sit on the edge with both hands on one side of your body, then pivot your body toward your hands as you slowly lower yourself into the water. When coming out of the pool, use the stairs again, if available. Otherwise, if the poolside ladder is painful or difficult to use, try stepping out using a collapsible, but sturdy, metal stepstool that rests solidly on the pool bottom.

Know when to quit. As with any exercise, you need to pay attention to your exertion in the water to keep from overdoing it. Sweat won't tell you you're working too hard. Neither will normal heart rate—your heart actually beats slower when your body is submerged, due in part to water pressure. But the most natural way to gauge intensity—perceived exertion—works just fine: If sucking air makes it tough to talk, take a breather. If you feel pained, persistently short of breath, dizzy, or disoriented, stop exercising and get out of the pool.

Gear for Wet Workouts

Theoretically, you don't need more than your own body to get a good workout in the water, but if you want to add resistance, ease, comfort, or safety, you might want to invest in some of the following items:

Water shoes. Whether it's an old pair of sneakers or special water shoes with nylon uppers and rubber soles, footwear provides traction underwater, prevents slipping on the poolside deck, and cushions your feet.

Foam noodles. You'll feel like a kid again while using these festive, flexible foam bars, but though they started as toys, exercise instructors use them both for resistance and as flotation devices.

Gloves and paddles. To add resistance beyond what you'd normally get with your hand, put on a pair of gloves with webbing between the fingers, or use paddles to push the water around.

Deep-water vest. Wear one of these close-fitting life jacket–like flotation devices to hold your face above water when you're in over your head, which frees you to concentrate on exercises such as running in place.

Water dumbbells. On land, these light-as-a-feather "weights" are worthless for building strength. Underwater, however, their buoyancy makes moving them a challenge for muscles.

Goggles. If you're not swimming with your head submerged, these may not be necessary, but some people find goggles protect sensitive eyes against chlorine irritation from treated pool water.

FINDING A WATER PROGRAM

Even if you have access to a private pool, it can be helpful to sign on with a water exercise program both for social camaraderie and guidance in your workout. You'll probably be able to find a program that suits your needs by checking:

> **the local YMCA or YWCA**

> **the Arthritis Foundation**

> **community centers in your neighborhood or town**

> **local colleges**

> **health clubs**

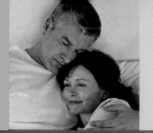

movement therapies: peace from the east

Some of the best forms of exercise are those in which your body moves naturally the way it does during everyday activities. But unless you make a conscious effort to move every part of your body, you may be letting some of your joints and muscles off the hook. Basic aerobic, strength, and flexibility exercises go a long way to making sure you work your entire body, but some people find value in going a step beyond—to movement disciplines that also nurture the mind and spirit.

Two of the best examples of movement methods are yoga and t'ai chi. Both involve moving your body into a series of stylized poses, and combine elements of both physical and mental discipline. While they have their origins in the East and sometimes invoke spiritual concepts, neither one is a religion—nor are they simply stretch routines. Yoga and t'ai chi do indeed enhance flexibility, but they also build strength, correct posture, may help relieve pain, and foster a sense of relaxation or peace of mind. At the same time, they're gentle enough that many moves can be practiced by people with arthritis.

Yoga: A Physical Philosophy

Yoga is an ancient practice going back thousands of years to India, where its methods were first written down by a Sanskrit scholar as far back as the second century B.C. In its purest form, yoga is a way of life that leads to physical and spiritual unity, assuming body and mind share powerful bonds and need to be balanced to achieve and maintain good health. On a pragmatic level, yoga integrates elements ranging from precise forms of exercise to personal ethics, diet, and other daily health habits.

Exercises are a key element of the overall discipline partly because performing slow and deliberate poses encourages you to focus on your body and become more attuned to it. Ultimately, the goal is to reach progressively higher states of enlightenment, but it's possible to gain benefits from yoga without striving for bliss.

One of the most popular forms is called hatha yoga, in which you practice physical poses known as *asanas* as a way of influencing the flow of life energy through the body. In yoga thinking, your breath is an outward sign of this life energy (known as *prana*), and deep breathing combined with meditation is central to proper practice. A complete routine is designed to work all parts of the body, stretching and toning muscles while improving range of motion in joints. While it's helpful to receive instruction, you don't need any special equipment to practice yoga—just a quiet room, a soft surface (exercises are usually done barefoot), and comfortable, lightweight clothes.

T'ai Chi: Slow-Motion Martial Art

Though its origins are in self-defense, the martial art known as t'ai chi chuan is actually a peaceful, gentle, and slow discipline that resembles dance more than combat. Like yoga, t'ai chi consists of postures or poses, which are performed in sequences (known as forms) that give t'ai chi a distinctively graceful, flowing quality. Here, too, the underlying philosophy is to promote the flow of life energy through the body and achieve physical, mental, and spiritual harmony. In traditional Chinese practice, t'ai chi is often done outdoors, to help connect the body's inner energy with the grander energy of the earth itself.

At the heart of t'ai chi are the twin concepts of yin and yang, contradictory yet complementary forces often represented with two merging semicircles of light and dark. In practice, t'ai chi is built on seemingly paradoxical ideas such as "alert relaxation" and "strength from softness." But there's nothing mysterious about the choreographed movements, which, beyond strength and flexibility, help promote coordination and balance.

It's possible to learn t'ai chi on your own with the help of instructional videos or books, but it's more useful (and easier) to learn from an instructor. Even "short" forms consist of up to 24 different movements that must be memorized, though actually performing the moves may take only 5 to 10 minutes. Longer forms contain more than 100 separate postures. Once you learn the moves, however, you can just as readily practice at home.

Identifying Instructors

Once considered esoteric, yoga and t'ai chi have adherents all across the country, and you're likely to find a class in your community. Due to yoga's popularity, you probably need look no further than the yellow pages, under "yoga instruction." If there's not a similar listing for t'ai chi, call the yoga establishments for referrals. Otherwise, try logging on to the T'ai Chi Network (www.taichinetwork.org), an Internet directory that you can search by hometown to find instructors in your area.

Science Weighs In

If concepts such as "life energy" and "harmony" strike you as overly mystical, you may prefer dwelling on the tangible benefits of yoga and t'ai chi. Though the research is sparse, a number of small studies suggest these disciplines have notable benefits for people with arthritis. For example, a recent study in India suggests that people with rheumatoid arthritis who practiced yoga were able to improve hand grip strength—unsurprising results, perhaps, from a "yoga research foundation." But the results mirror those of a University of Pennsylvania study seven years earlier, which found that eight weeks of yoga helped osteoarthritis patients significantly improve finger range of motion, tenderness, and pain compared with patients who did no yoga.

One of the few studies ever done on the effects of t'ai chi on arthritis was presented to a recent meeting of the American College of Rheumatology. Chinese researchers found that older osteoarthritis patients who took a 12-week t'ai chi program showed significant improvement in physical function, muscle strength, balance, and pain compared with a control group.

YOGA TIPS FOR PEOPLE WITH ARTHRITIS

> Though yoga is considered an individual discipline, the American Yoga Association suggests that people with arthritis make yoga classes part of an overall self-management program. Yoga classes provide instruction, impose structure on your daily practicing, and help you connect with other people.

> If you find that stiff or painful joints limit your motion during yoga, try heating the affected areas with a heating pad or perhaps a hot bath before doing your routine. Caution: If joints are acutely inflamed, check with your doctor about whether heat treatment is appropriate.

> To get the most out of yoga, practitioners say it's best to do a daily routine. You don't need large amounts of time, but you should strive for a session of about 30 minutes, perhaps with 15 minutes of exercise and 15 minutes of breathing and meditation.

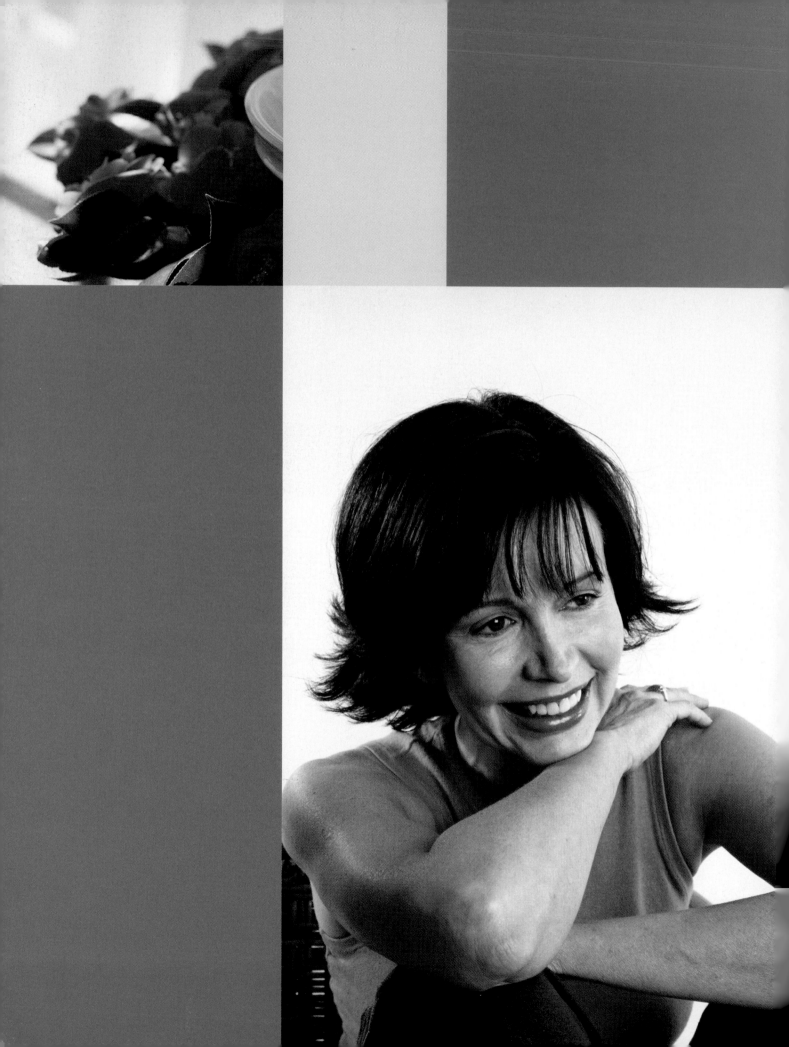

targeted exercises

The pages ahead may seem intimidating, even frightening. All these exercises! So much instruction! If this was your reaction, it's time for a change of attitude. Think of this part like a cook-book: a wonderful array of healthy movements to browse and sample, none mandatory but all good for you. ● When you look closely, you'll discover that these stretches, exercises, and massages are simple, gentle, and natural – perfect for people with arthritis! So give them a try. Then, in Part Four, we'll show you how to put them together into the perfect regular routine.

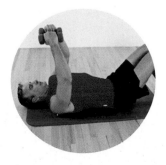

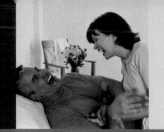
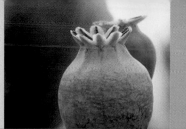

getting into action

Think of Part One of this book as "ready," Part Two as "set." Now you're at "go!" It is time for you to get moving. In the pages ahead, you will discover a broad range of stretches, strengthening moves, and massages, most of them quite unlike what you would find in more general fitness books. The differences? First, they are gentler and more natural movements. Second, they were chosen as much for their beneficial effects for joints as for their effectiveness in building muscle.

Maybe you already do simple range-of-motion exercises or take strolls around your neighborhood fairly regularly. That puts you ahead of the game. What happens next is not a race, but a journey. There's nobody to beat and you don't have to push yourself too hard. Comfortable progress, week by week, will move you toward your beginning goals. Then you'll be able to establish new goals that you could not even have imagined at the start.

The exercises in this section are the key to your success in fighting pain and getting fit. Each is explained step by step, with plenty of tips and secrets from some of the nation's best experts on making exercise work for people with arthritis. Not every exercise will be right for you. Start by establishing your level of physical function using the self-scoring questions on page 39. If you already know at which level you should begin, use the reminder chart "Figuring Your Function Level" to establish the starting parameters for your program. Keep in mind that these guidelines are starting points, and are deliberately on the conservative side. The last thing you need is an exercise program that causes more pain. But even after one or two workouts, you'll have a sense of whether you can handle more. If you're comfortable taking on harder exercises without causing significant discomfort, feel free to do more repetitions, stretch longer, choose more challenging movements, or add time to your cardio workout.

Once you get started with a program, you'll quickly become comfortable with the motions your exercises require. In many cases, it's possible for simple modifications to make the exercises you're doing more challenging as you get more fit, so you don't have to change a routine you already like. At the same time, if you want to move on to new exercises or add elements to your workout, you'll find options for doing so.

The Parts and the Whole

Bodybuilders and serious fitness enthusiasts love to talk about "isolating" muscles—doing exercises that concentrate on a single muscle that will produce just the right ripple to enhance the exerciser's buff beauty. Your goals are more pragmatic. When you strive to improve function, isolating muscles can indeed build strength in critical areas that support arthritic joints. But it's just as important to make muscles work together. That, after all, is how the body operates in real life.

Physiologists think of the body as a mechanical system of many segments in which forces applied to one joint can cause a chain reaction of effects in other joints through the levers of the skeleton and the muscles. (They call it the kinetic chain.) Sometimes these effects can be predicted. For example, if you have arthritis in one knee, the way you move your body to compensate raises your risk of arthritis in the opposite knee and hip.

Bottom line: Physiologists say that in addition to exercises that work specific muscles, it's important to do exercises or activities that work bones, joints, and muscles in ways they actually function in day-to-day activities such as climbing stairs or getting out of a chair. And if you have arthritis in the knee, don't just work to strengthen muscles supporting that joint, but build strength throughout the rest of your body as well. "Everything is connected to everything else," says Virginia Kraus, M.D., Ph.D., medical director of the Arthritis Rehabilitation Program at Duke University Center for Living. "So it's important to do a variety of exercises, such as aerobic walking in addition to a range of strength exercises."

That's an important message. While the pages ahead are organized by the joints of the body, don't limit yourself to the exercises targeted at your problem spot. Indeed, as important as it is to learn these exercises properly, it is just as important to learn how to put them together into a sequence that is absolutely best for you and your needs. That is what Part Four is all about. By using these two sections together, you have the ultimate resource for exercising away arthritis pain.

Figuring Your Function Level

Whatever your level of function, you'll find exercises in this section that you can do without causing further pain. Follow the guidelines below to decide which exercises are appropriate for your function level. To determine what level you should start with, take the self-scoring quiz on page 39. And don't forget to make aerobic exercise a part of your routine!

LEVEL 1

Low Physical Function

- **Flexibility:** Hold stretches for 15 seconds
- **Strength:** 1 set of 6 repetitions with an easy weight, two to three days a week.
- **Aerobics:** 5 minutes a day, three to five days a week

LEVEL 2

Moderate Physical Function

- **Flexibility:** Hold stretches for 20 seconds
- **Strength:** 1 set of 6 to 8 repetitions with an easy weight, two to three days a week
- **Aerobics:** 10 to 12 minutes a day, three to five days a week

LEVEL 3

Good Physical Function

- **Flexibility:** Hold stretches for 30 seconds
- **Strength:** 1 set of 8 repetitions with a moderate weight, two to three days a week
- **Aerobics:** 20 minutes a day, three to five days a week

Modifying Your Program

Everybody has good days and bad. But some bad days are worse than others. How should you change—not abandon—your exercise program in response to flare-ups of pain or the draggy torpor of fatigue? Score your responses to the following questions and adjust your program as suggested below.

How much pain do you have today?

NONE	0
VERY MILD	1
MILD	2
MODERATE	3
SEVERE	4
WORST	5

How much fatigue do you have today?

NONE	0
VERY MILD	1
MILD	2
MODERATE	3
SEVERE	4
WORST	5

Scoring

With pain or fatigue scores of:

0–2 > Proceed as planned with your exercise program, gradually increasing intensity as improvements in your fitness and function allow.

3 > Exercise at the same level as the previous session (without adding resistance or intensity), if you exercised within the past week.

4 > Reduce the number of repetitions of strength exercises and aerobic time by 50 percent.

5 > It may be best not to do your regular exercise routine today. But try to do some simple, gentle body movements throughout the day, perhaps after taking a warm bath or shower.

The knees and hips are the body's main weight-bearing joints, subject to enormous stress from daily activities. Just stepping up a single stair, for example, puts hundreds of pounds of pressure on lower-body joints and the muscles that support them. You can't do much to make your joints more durable, but making your muscles stronger lets them take on more of the load, relieving your knees and hips.

"Muscles of hips and knees are critical for mobility and everyday function, whether you're taking the stairs, getting out of a car, or lifting laundry or groceries," says Daniel Rooks, Ph.D., director of the Be Well! Tanger Center for Health Management at Harvard's Beth Israel Deaconess Medical Center. "They often work together, so you want a mix of exercises that strengthen multiple muscles together along with exercises that work muscles supporting the joints separately."

STRETCHES

Wall Sit

This is a gentle move to stretch stiff hamstrings at the back of the leg.

1. Sit on the floor, back against a wall, knees bent and heels, hip-width apart, planted two feet in front of you. Your toes should point upward at a 45-degree angle.

2. Slowly slide or walk your heels forward so that your knees get closer to the ground until you feel a slight stretch at the back of your knees **a**. Relax your muscles and hold this position.

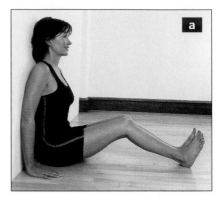

TIP: Pressing your back against the wall keeps your pelvis fixed so that all movement is concentrated on your hamstrings.

Seated Knee Extension

This is a good stretch and warmup for a strength exercise, since it uses the same basic motion with weights. You need a chair high enough to slightly elevate your heels off the floor. To give a regular chair extra height, use cushions.

1. Sit in a chair, back straight, both feet flat on the floor, and knees bent 90 degrees.

2. Slowly straighten your right knee as far as you comfortably can, so that toes point toward the ceiling **a**. Hold. Repeat with the other leg.

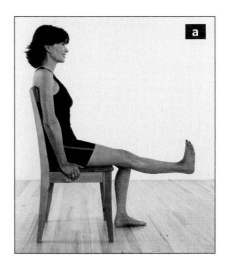

TIP: Keep your spine pressed against the back of the chair so that you don't arch your back. If the quadriceps muscles at the front of your thighs are weak, this movement will help strengthen them while also stretching your hamstrings.

Straight-Leg Stretch

If you can sit and straighten your legs in front of you, try this more advanced stretch.

1. Sit on the floor, legs extended straight in front of you, toes pointed toward the ceiling. Keep your back straight and your hands resting on the outside of your thighs.

2. Slide your hands forward along your legs toward your toes, reaching as far as you comfortably can and putting your chest as close to your knees as possible **a**. Hold for a gentle stretch at the back of your legs.

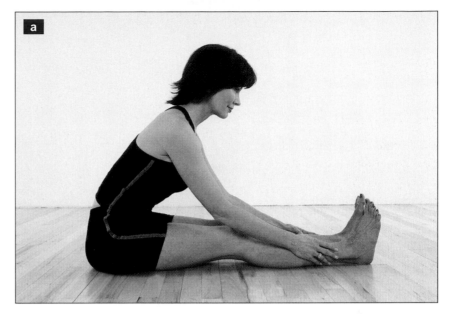

TIP: Don't arch your back during the stretch: A straight spine protects the back and allows a better stretch of your hamstrings. You don't have to reach your toes: As you become more limber, you'll be able to reach farther.

Seated V

This exercise lengthens the adductor muscles of the groin area in the inner thigh as well as the hamstrings—a twist allows you to stretch both sets of muscles.

1. Sit on the floor, back straight, legs extended, toes pointed toward the ceiling, and feet spread comfortably apart in a V. Hands should rest in front of you between your thighs **a**.

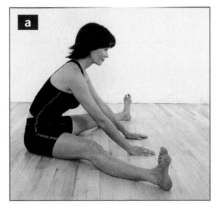

2. Keeping your back straight, gently "walk" your hands out in front of you until you feel a slight stretch in your inner thighs **b**. Hold.

TIP: Use this position for a hamstring stretch by putting your left hand on the inside of your right thigh and the right hand on the outside, then moving both hands down your right leg. Hold and repeat on the left leg.

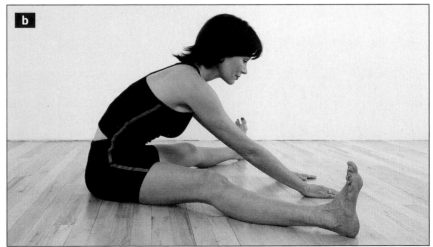

Standing Quad Stretch

Top athletes use this stretch for lengthening the all-important quadriceps muscle on the front of the thigh.

1. Stand with feet about hip-width apart, holding on to a chair or counter with your left hand.

2. Standing on your left leg with the knee slightly flexed, bend your right knee so that your foot is behind you. Keeping your knees next to each other, gently bring your right heel toward your buttocks.

Grab your right foot with your right hand 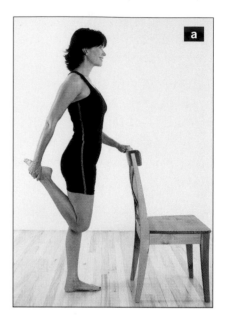. Hold.

3. Let your right foot down and repeat with your left leg.

TIP: Keep your knees close together during the stretch. If muscles are tight, you'll tend to move at the hip rather than the knee, which changes the stretch. If you have trouble balancing or experience pain standing on one leg, you can perform this same move while lying on your stomach.

Lying Quad and Hip Stretch

Similar to the standing quad stretch, this exercise works both the quadriceps and the hip flexor muscles, prime movers in the torso.

1. Lie on your left side, using your left arm as a pillow to support your head. Bend your left hip (which is resting on the floor) to a 90-degree angle so that your knee is in front of you 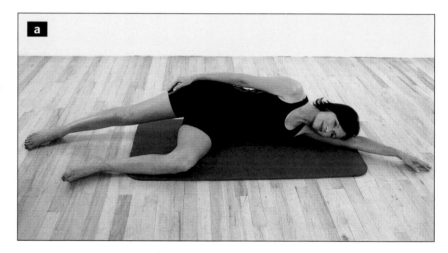.

2. Bend your top (right) knee to a 90-degrees angle, grabbing your right ankle with your right hand and bringing the heel back toward the buttocks 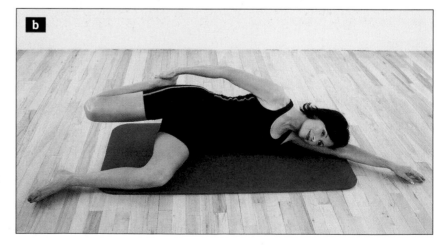. Hold. Repeat with the other leg.

TIP: Don't straighten your bottom knee. Keeping the knee bent helps fix the pelvis in a slightly forward position that provides a better hip stretch when you move the top leg back.

Lying Pelvis Rotation

This simple move uses gravity to stretch the abductor muscles on the outside of the hip.

1. Lie on your right side, using your right arm as a pillow to support your head. Keeping your right leg straight, bend your left hip at a 90-degree angle so your knee is in front of you.

2. Relax the muscles of your left leg so that your left knee slowly drops toward the ground to produce a gentle rotational stretch of the hip 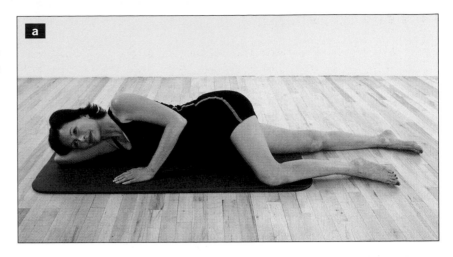. Stay relaxed and hold. Repeat with the other leg.

TIP: Start with the lying pelvis rotation if your hip muscles are tight. When you're more limber, try a variation: Lie on your back with feet flat on floor so your knees are pointing toward the ceiling. Keeping shoulders on the ground, slowly lower both knees to the right to get a stretch in left hip and buttocks. Hold, return to the starting position, and repeat on the other side.

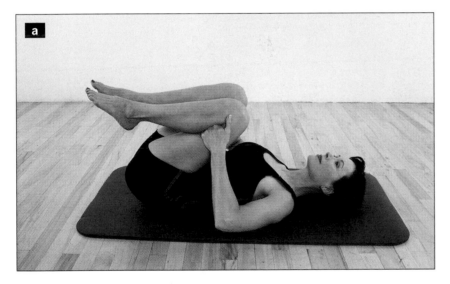

Knees to Chest

A classic for easing low back discomfort, this stretch can be done lying on a bed and also helps your hips and knees.

1. Lie on your back with legs relaxed and straight, toes pointing toward the ceiling.

2. Put your hands on the back of your thighs under your knees and smoothly pull both knees as far toward your shoulders as is comfortable to stretch the extensor muscles at the back of the hips in the buttocks area 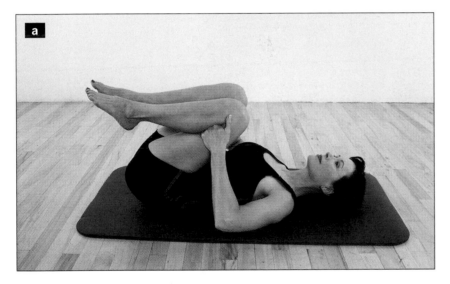. Hold.

everyday *secrets*

Wide-ranging advice for better fitness, more movement, and safer exercise for people with arthritis.

Keep eyes open. You may be tempted to close your eyes during exercise so you can concentrate on your muscles or breathing. Don't. Balance relies on visual input to the brain; keep your eyes open to steady yourself.

Spread correctly. Many exercise guides tell you to start standing exercises with your feet shoulder-width apart. If you have arthritis, plant your feet hip-width apart. This narrower distance puts your knees, hips, and feet in alignment for good posture and improved biomechanics.

Keep support nearby. During standing exercises, use—or keep within easy grasp—a sturdy chair, countertop, or even wall, to maintain your balance and reduce the risk of injury.

Build abs with reps. The abdominal exercises in this book don't use weights, so when you master the most difficult version of a given exercise, how do you top that? Try to add a repetition at least every other time you do the exercise.

continued on page 60

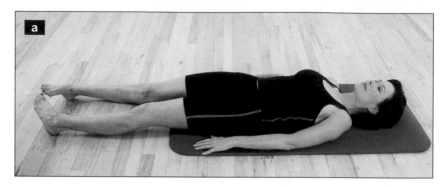

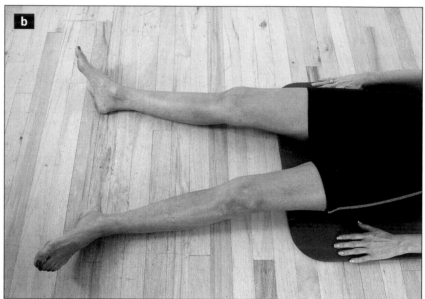

Leg Twist

Another comfortable stretch that can be done in bed, this windshield wiper motion stretches the hip rotator muscles, which helps hip mobility and may help ease pain from sciatica.

1. Lie on your back with feet about shoulder-width apart, toes pointed toward the ceiling.

2. Smoothly rotate your ankles to first roll your toes toward each other **a**. Hold. Now rotate ankles to roll toes away from each other **b** . Hold.

TIP: You don't have to be lying down to do this stretch. Performed while sitting on the floor, it's particularly effective when done from the seated V position.

STRENGTH EXERCISES

`LEVEL 1`

Partial Squat

Squats build strength on all sides of your upper legs and buttocks, supporting a wide variety of everyday activities. If you experience knee pain, start with this mild version.

1. Stand with feet about hip-width apart, touching a chair or counter for balance.

2. Keeping your back straight and your eyes looking forward, slowly lower your body as if you were going to sit in a chair **a**. Stop when you reach a point halfway to a sitting position, then raise yourself back to a standing position.

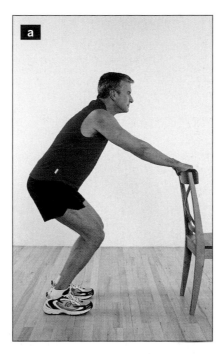

TIP: Your legs should do the work. Use the chair or countertop only to keep your balance, not to support your weight. Try to do the exercise hands-free. To keep your body properly aligned, think about pushing down with your heels. Don't let your knees move forward of your toes.

NOTCH IT UP: Lower yourself all the way to a chair. From the same starting position, sit lightly on the front half of a chair, then immediately stand up again.

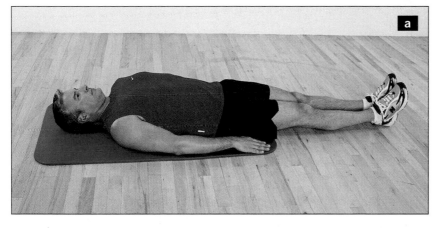

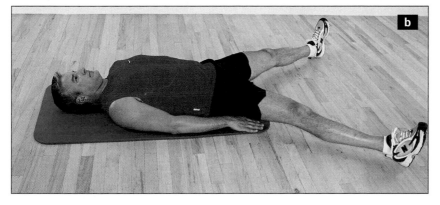

Lying Hip Abduction

Like the leg part of making snow angels (only you're warm and dry), this exercise works the abductor muscles at the outside of the hip.

1. Lie on your back with your feet pointing toward the ceiling and your legs together **a**.

2. Keeping your legs straight, move your feet comfortably apart and bring them back together again **b**.

TIP: Do this gently and slowly, pausing at the full extension. A fast scissoring motion isn't as safe or as beneficial for your muscles.

Heel Slide

This simple exercise with two variations works the hamstring muscles.

1. Lie on your back with your legs straight and your toes pointed toward the ceiling **a**.

2. Keeping your left leg straight, slowly bend your right leg so your knee moves toward the ceiling and your heel slides toward your buttocks **b**.

3. Slide your heel back to the starting position. After one set, repeat with the other leg.

NOTCH IT UP: Start by doing one leg at a time. As you gain strength, do both legs together, which is more difficult.

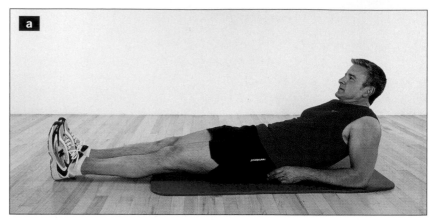

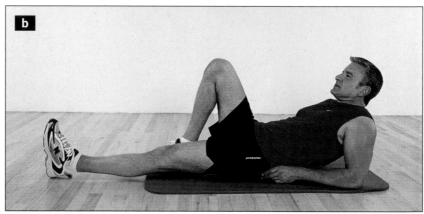

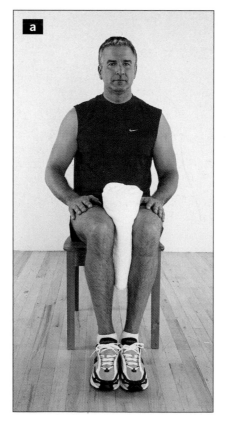

Towel Squeeze

This is an isometric exercise that safely works the muscles of the inner thigh, which help stabilize the knees and hips.

1. Sit in a chair with a large, rolled-up bath towel placed between your knees and thighs.

2. Gently squeeze your knees together as firmly as you comfortably can **a**. Hold for six seconds to do one repetition.

TIP: Don't worry if your knees touch as long as the contact doesn't cause pain: The towel is meant to cushion knees, not separate them. If you prefer, you can also use a folded bed pillow or a small sofa pillow.

Lower-Body Extension

Though this exercise by itself provides a good workout for the hips, a more advanced version in level 2, the Bird Dog, offers a combined move that also targets the upper body.

1. Get down on your hands and knees on the floor, a rug, or an exercise mat.

2. Extend your right leg out behind you, keeping your foot about one inch off the floor as you straighten your knee 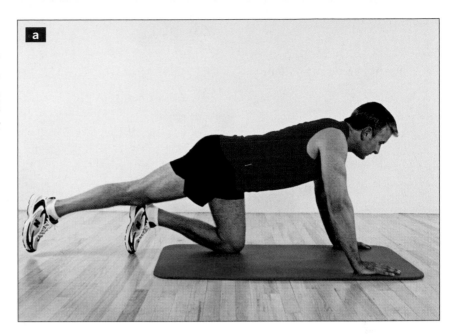. Return to the starting position and repeat with the other leg to complete one repetition. Continue alternating legs until you finish a set.

Lying Hip Extension

This exercise works large muscles in the hips and buttocks as well as the hamstrings, which stabilize the hips and help walking and sitting.

1. Lie on your stomach with your legs straight and your toes pointed down. You can prop your upper body on your elbows, but may find it more relaxing to lie flat, supporting your head with your arms or hands.

2. Keeping your knee straight, lift your entire right leg so that your foot is one to two inches off the floor 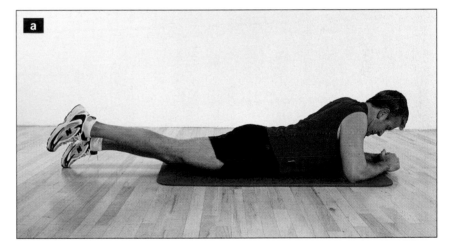. Lower your leg back to the floor.

3. Repeat with the other leg. This is one repetition.

TIP: Keep your body stable and relaxed so that all movement is concentrated at the hip joint.

NOTCH IT UP: As you become stronger, you can make this exercise more intense by doing extra repetitions or adding strap-on ankle weights.

everyday
secrets

Know which side. If pain or decreased range of motion makes walking difficult, use a cane or rolling walker in the hand opposite the painful knee or hip.

Consider a splint. If overzealous exercising makes joint pain flare up, give the injured area a rest. A splint will temporarily stabilize the joint and keep you from hurting it further. You can buy splints over the counter at a drugstore or get them fitted by an occupational therapist. You can buy splints for fingers, hands, wrists, elbows, knees, and ankles.

Know the limits. If you've had total hip or knee replacement, check with your doctor before doing any exercises. These procedures eliminate certain moves from your repertoire for at least two to six months after surgery. You should, for example, avoid exercises that involve high-impact stress on the lower extremities, leg adduction (moving legs inward against resistance), or flexing the new joint beyond 90 degrees.

continued on page 64

LEVEL 2

Standing Hip Extension

A standing version of the lying hip extension in level 1 (page 59), this exercise provides a more intense workout for the hips, buttocks, hamstrings, and lower back.

1. Stand with feet about hip-width apart, lightly holding a chair or counter.

2. Without bending the knee, move your right leg from the hip back behind you **a**. Return slowly to the starting position. After one set, repeat with the other leg.

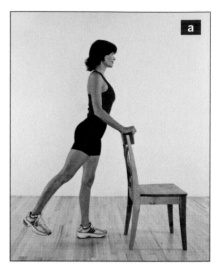

TIPS: Don't lock the knee of the leg you stand on, but instead keep it slightly bent. While the motion is pendulum-like, you shouldn't let momentum do the work. Perform the move slowly, especially during the return phase.

Standing Knee Flexion

A tandem exercise to the seated knee extension (page 62), this move strengthens the hamstrings at the back of the thigh.

1. Wearing ankle weights, stand behind a chair with feet about hip-width apart, holding on to the back of the chair.

2. Smoothly bend your left knee, drawing your heel toward your buttocks **a**, then slowly return your foot to the ground. After one set, repeat with the other leg.

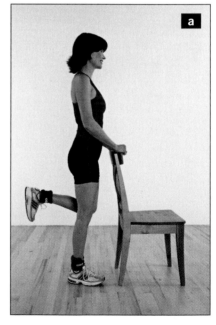

TIPS:
• Start with enough weight to allow you to comfortably do the 6 to 8 repetitions suggested for level 2 exercises.

• Keep your knees next to each other as you bend your knee so that your upper legs remain parallel.

• Start by raising your heel so that your lower leg is parallel to the floor. As you become more conditioned, lift your heel closer to your buttocks. Add weight as you gain strength.

Side Hip Abduction

This simple exercise works the ab–ductor muscles on the outside of the hip and outer thigh.

1. Lie on your left side with both legs extended and resting one on top of the other, supporting your head with your left hand.

2. In a smooth and controlled mo–tion, lift your fully extended right leg straight up as high as you com–fortably can 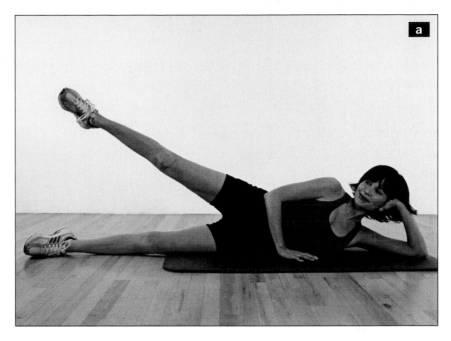. Then lower it back to the starting position. After one set, repeat with the other leg.

TIP: If you feel unstable in the starting position, try bending the lower leg to provide a wider base of support.

Stair Step-Up

Easily a part of any exercise routine, the step-up can be modified in a variety of ways to make it more challenging as you progress.

1. Stand in front of a step with both feet on the floor about hip-width apart.

2. Place your right foot solidly on the stair and step up **a**. Bring your left foot up and touch it lightly on the step before lowering it back to the floor **b**.

3. Step down with your right foot.

4. Step up with your left foot, bringing your right foot up and touching it lightly on the step, then lowering it back to the floor. Alter-nate steps in this way, counting one repetition when each foot has stepped up one time.

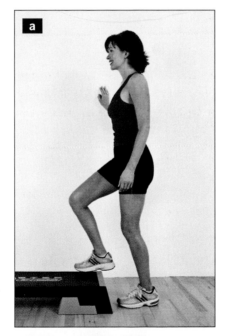

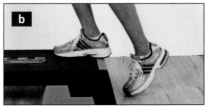

TIP: To keep track of repetitions, count step-ups on just one foot. Though you can use a special exercise step for this move, it's not necessary. In fact, a regu-lar step in your home may be preferable because you can lightly grasp the stair rail for support.

NOTCH IT UP: The first way to make this exercise more difficult is to do a set using only one foot instead of alternat-ing. For example, use the right foot to step up, step down, then step up again rather than alternating with the left foot. When you've finished a set of step-ups with the right foot, do a set with the left. A second way to make this ex-ercise more difficult is to alternate your feet, but raise yourself up two steps at a time instead of just one.

Seated Knee Extension with Weight

Adding ankle weights to this stretch (p.52) makes it a muscle-building exercise for the quadriceps at the front of the thigh.

1. Strap weights around your ankles. Sit in a chair, back straight, both feet flat on the floor, and knees bent at 90 degrees.

2. Slowly straighten your right knee as far as you comfortably can, lifting your weighted foot so that toes point toward the ceiling 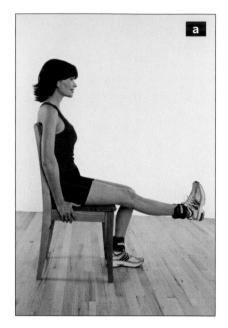. Smoothly lower your foot to the starting position.

3. After one set, repeat with the other leg.

TIPS:

• Sit back in the chair so your back is straight and well supported. The seat of the chair should support your thighs and the back of your knees. To make the chair high enough for full range of motion, sit on a cushion.

• Start with enough weight to allow you to comfortably do the 6 to 8 repetitions suggested for level 2 exercises. Add weight as you gain strength.

Bird Dog

Building on the hip extension (page 59), this exercise not only works muscles of the hips, but also the back, chest, shoulders, and arms. Its multi-element motion improves balance and coordination, and helps promote good posture.

1. Get down on your hands and knees on the floor, a rug, or an exercise mat.

2. Extend your left leg out behind you, keeping your foot about one to two inches off the floor as you straighten your knee.

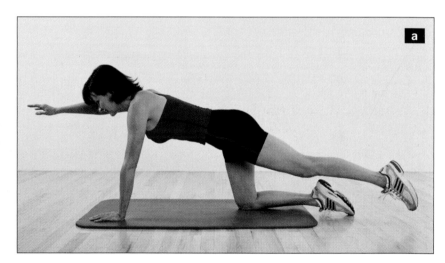

3. At the same time you extend your left leg, reach out straight in front of you with your right arm 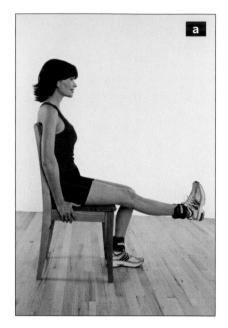. Return to the starting position and repeat with the other leg and arm to complete one repetition.

4. Continue alternating legs and arms until you finish a set.

TIP: Try to keep your back as flat as possible during the movement.

LEVEL 3

Ball Squat

You will need a large exercise ball for this squat, which works your thighs in the same way conventional squats do. This is more challenging, however, because it forces you to keep yourself steady against an uneven surface, which promotes good balance.

1. Stand next to a wall with your feet hip-width apart. Put the exercise ball on your lower back between you and the wall, holding the ball in place with your body.

2. Slowly bending your knees, lower yourself until your thighs are parallel to the floor, allowing the

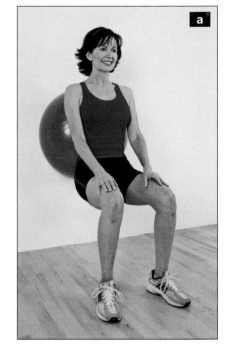

ball to roll behind your back as your body drops **a**. Slowly straighten your legs and roll the ball back to the starting position.

TIP: As in a regular squat, your knees should be aligned with your feet. Don't place your feet in front of your body to lean back harder against the ball. If pain prevents you from bending your knees to 90 degrees, lower yourself to a point that's comfortable and gradually expand your range as you get stronger.

NOTCH IT UP: If your knee comfort allows, you can give thigh muscles a vigorous isometric workout by holding your body in place for a count of 1 to 3 in the lowered position.

Side Thrust Kick

This exercise provides a good workout for the muscles that surround the hip while also expanding the knees' range of motion.

1. Lie on your right side with both legs extended and your head propped on your right hand. Bring your upper (left) leg forward so that your left knee is in front of your hip, with the knee bent to a 90-degree angle **a**.

2. Kick your left foot out at a 45-degree angle from the floor, straightening your leg as you kick **b**. Lower your foot and return your left leg to its straightened starting position. After one set, repeat with the other leg.

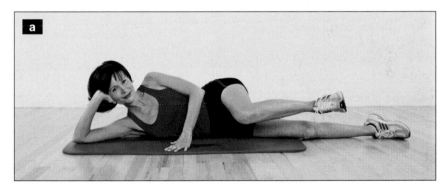

TIP: When pressing your leg upward, imagine you're kicking a spot about three feet in front of you.

NOTCH IT UP: Bend the upper leg at an angle sharper than 90 degrees so that your upper foot is closer to the knee of the lower leg.

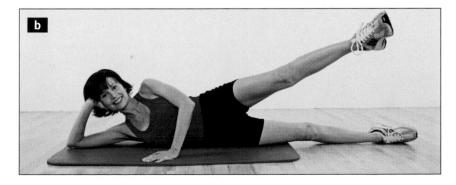

everyday
secrets

Use good gear. Theoretically, anything heavy can be used for resistance exercises—milk jugs filled with sand or bags of rice. Such ad hoc gear may keep your equipment costs down, but most resistance exercises are more effective, more comfortable, and safer if you use equipment designed for fitness use.

Do it softly and twice. If you find a particular stretch difficult, don't push it. Instead, do the stretch as well as you can twice, resting in between. The repeated lengthening of your muscles will provide an extra degree of flexibility.

Add sets, not weights. A more intense exercise is usually taken to mean one involving heavier weights. But the issue is the overall volume of exercise, not just the weight of resistance. If you want to make an exercise more intense but find additional resistance to be uncomfortable, you can add sets or repetitions for an extra challenge.

continued on page 72

Partial Stationary Lunge

The lunge is a time-tested exercise that really builds up the muscles involved with walking, climbing stairs, and getting out of a chair.

1. Take a larger-than-normal step forward with your right foot. This is your starting position, and you'll keep both feet planted through your repetitions **a**.

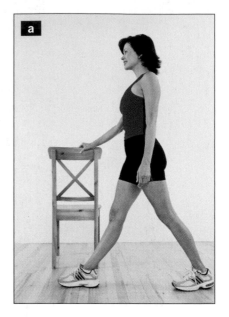

2. Keeping your upper body straight, bend your right knee and slide your pelvis forward until your knee is over the toe of your right foot **b**. The heel of your left foot will come off the floor. To further lower your body, bend your left knee.

3. Return to the starting position and repeat on the same side. After one set, do the same with the other leg.

TIP: The difficulty of this move can be adjusted by the size of your starting step: Every increase of distance intensifies resistance. When you can do 12 repetitions comfortably, extend your first step another half foot. If needed, use a chair or counter to keep your balance, but not to support your weight.

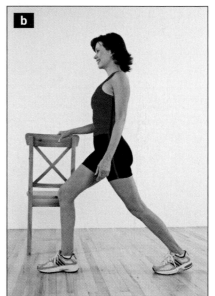

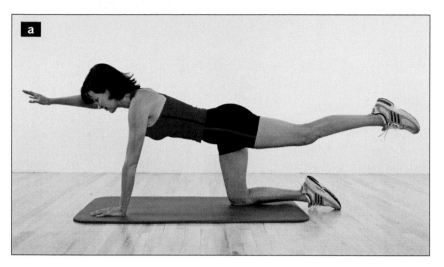

Advanced Bird Dog

Building on the basic bird dog move in level 2, this more advanced exercise not only works muscles of the hips, but also the back and shoulders.

1. Get down on your hands and knees on the floor, a rug, or an exercise mat.

2. Extend your left leg out behind you, raising your foot so that your entire leg is parallel to the floor—a more strenuous position than in the basic bird dog. At the same time, reach out straight in front of you with your right arm **a** .

3. Return to the starting position and repeat with the other leg and arm to complete one repetition. Continue alternating legs and arms until you finish a set.

AT THE *Fitness Center*

If you have access to good-quality exercise machines, here's what to use for your knees and hips:

LEG PRESS

There are many types of leg press machines, but with the best units for people with arthritis, extending your legs during the lift moves the seat, not the foot plate. This prevents uneven or sudden pressure on knees if you perform the exercise too quickly. With machines that move the foot plate, you must keep movements slow and controlled. Machines with reclining seats in which your body forms a V are most comfortable. Machines in which you lie flat with feet directly overhead are difficult to get in and out of.

KNEE EXTENSION

You have unlimited resistance variations with a machine to do this exercise for your quadriceps. Although this exercise can be done one leg at a time (especially during rehabilitation), doing both legs at once promotes muscle balance by encouraging both sides of the body to work together like they do in daily life.

KNEE FLEXION

This is often a tandem exercise with the knee extension, designed to work your hamstrings. You may find older versions of this machine in which you do the exercise lying down. These machines work well, but you'll find a seated machine easier to mount and dismount.

MACHINE ABDUCTION/ ADDUCTION

Machines are a great way to isolate the muscles at the sides of your upper leg. If your gym doesn't have a single machine that does both abduction and adduction, it should have separate machines for doing these same movements. When beginning with a machine, use the same resistance for both abduction and adduction.

MASSAGES

Hip Circle

This gentle massage helps boost circulation in the hip.

1. Before you start, place your hands on your hips and hold for a moment, then begin rubbing your palms over the sides of your hips in large circles to improve circulation close to the surface of the skin **a**.

2. Resting your thumb on your waist for support, use your fingers to press firmly on the side of your hip **b**. Move your fingers in a circular motion to stimulate blood flow deeper in the muscle.

Kneecap Squeeze

This massage expels fluid from the knee joint when you squeeze, but allows it to flow back more abundantly when you release, giving some relief from pain.

1. Sit in a chair and place your right hand over your right knee so that your palm is covering your kneecap.

2. Use your fingers and thumb to squeeze the sides of your kneecap **a**. Hold the squeeze for about two seconds, then release. Repeat on the left knee.

Knee Orbit

A thorough workover relaxes the knee joint.

1. Sit in a chair and place your right hand over your right knee. Find the edge of your kneecap with your fingers, then gently massage with small, circular motions **a**.

2. Continue massaging as you move your fingers around the entire perimeter of the kneecap **b**. Include the top area where thigh muscles attach to the kneecap **c**. Continue the massage for one to two minutes, then repeat on the left knee.

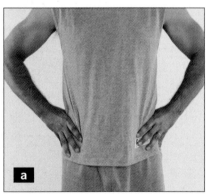

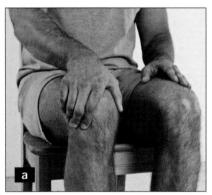

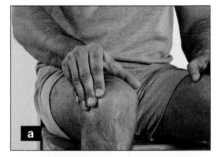

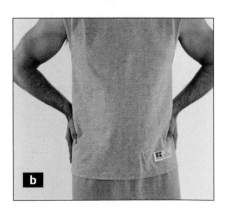

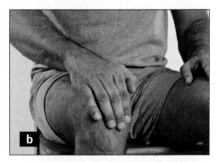

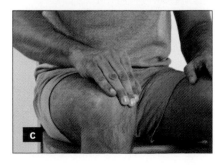

12 Ways to Walk More

You exercise your hips and knees so you can walk more, without pain or exhaustion. But doctors will also tell you that the best way to walk more is to … walk more. Here are 12 ideas to get you on your feet and moving:

1. Every night, immediately after dinner, take a 20-minute stroll. Don't let the weather stop you—that's what jackets, boots, and umbrellas are for. Indeed, there's something wonderfully refreshing and childlike about a walk in the rain or snow. Post-dinner is the perfect time for a walk. It gets you away from the television, it's when others are outside, it's a lovely time of day, and it stops you from eating more.

2. Develop a habit: Never sit while talking on the phone. Instead, walk around your home if you have a portable phone, and if not, pace back and forth. You'd be surprised how much movement you can do when you are concentrating on a conversation rather than the exertion.

3. Make more social events around walking. For example, rather than meeting friends for coffee or lunch, suggest meeting at the public gardens for a stroll.

4. When watching television, always get up and move about during commercials. You've seen them already, anyhow. During a single one-hour show, you can get in more than 10 minutes of activity!

5. Take the stairs, take the stairs, take the stairs. You've heard it a million times, but if it is three flights or less, you have no excuse to take an elevator, unless your arthritis pain is truly prohibitive. In that case, take one flight of stairs instead.

6. For an evening's diversion, do some outdoor window-shopping. Strolling down a street of shops is great for people-watching, talking, and feeling alive.

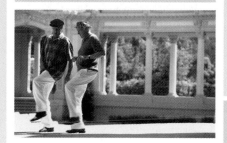

7. Split your lunch hour in two: 30 minutes of eating, 30 minutes of walking. No one needs to eat for 60 minutes. Chances are, you're just sitting and talking. Invite your lunch partner along for the stroll.

8. Find a park or a wilderness area near you and commit to a nature walk a few times a week. Nothing lifts your soul as much as a good walk in the woods (or by the lake, or even in the desert).

9. Locate the outdoor mailbox closest to your home, and get in the habit of walking to it to send off your bills or letters. Maybe it'll get you to write more letters—wonderful for your hands, even better for your friends and family.

10. If you have little children in your life—be they yours, grandchildren, nieces, nephews, or even just neighbors—commit to the following per year: a trip to the ball game, a trip to the circus, a trip to the zoo, a trip to the aquarium, a trip to the kids' museum. Buy the tickets long in advance, and exercise in advance so you're ready for a full day of fun.

11. Somehow, somehow, find a way to dance. Don't wait for a date or a wedding. Turn on the stereo and dance at home. Join a square-dance group or take ballroom lessons.

12. Come up with a personal "instant walk" trigger. For example, anytime you become drowsy, take a five-minute walk. Or, anytime you want a snack. Or, anytime you get angry, bored, melancholy, or stressed. Walking isn't just an antidote for arthritis pain, it is a wonderful way to work out mental and emotional issues as well.

Shoulders help you maintain good posture and are critical for daily tasks ranging from carrying a bag of topsoil, picking a book off a shelf over your head, or hoisting yourself out of a chair. Their wide range of motion makes strong shoulders essential to every upper-arm movement—forward, back, up, down, side to side. Their versatility also makes shoulders easy to injure, but you can protect them by making supporting muscles stronger. Here are 7 stretches and 10 exercises to do just that.

STRETCHES

Shoulder Roll

This stretch is helpful for people who hold muscle tension in the neck or upper back.

1. Stand up straight with feet hip-width apart and knees slightly bent. Relax your shoulders **a**. With arms down by your side, move your shoulders forward to stretch your shoulder blades, shrugging them toward your ears **b**. Move them backward so shoulder blades squeeze together, and return to the starting position for a full backward circle. Do 6 repetitions.

2. From the starting position, repeat the exercise in the opposite direction, moving your shoulders back, up toward your ears in a shrugging motion, forward, then back down to the starting position, making a full forward circle.

TIP: Try to move in a smooth, continuous circular motion, making movements as large as is comfortable. Start with small circles, and over time, try to make your circles bigger.

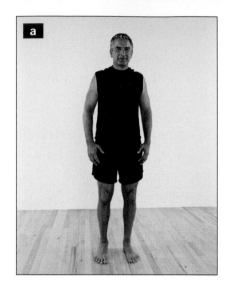

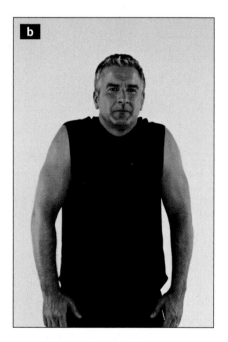

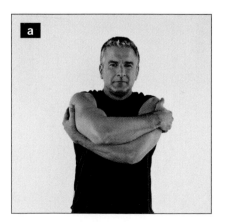

Self-Hug

1. Stand up straight with your feet hip-width apart and your knees slightly bent.

2. Wrap your arms around yourself, reaching each hand to grasp the opposite shoulder or the side of your torso to produce a stretch in the back of the shoulders. Hold.

Knuckle Rub

1. Stand up straight with feet hip-width apart and knees slightly bent, hands down by your side. Make a fist and, with knuckles facing forward, move your hands behind you and place your knuckles against your lower back.

2. Gently move your knuckles up your back until you feel a stretch in the front part of your shoulder and your upper arms **a** . Hold.

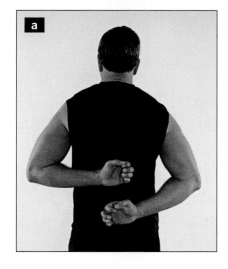
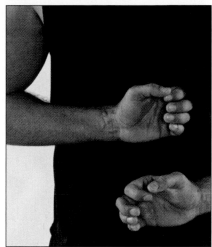

Wall Climb

This combination exercise stretches the shoulders in two directions, and is especially good for people with a restricted range of shoulder motion. It also provides a workout for your fingers.

1. Stand up straight facing a wall from 18 inches away, with your feet hip-width apart, knees slightly bent, and arms hanging down by your side.

2. Reach out with both arms and touch the wall at about waist level **a** . Use your fingers like spiders' legs to climb the wall until you feel a stretch at the back and sides of your shoulders. Hold. Slowly "climb" your fingers back down to waist level.

3. Turn so that your right hip is facing the wall from the same distance away **b** . Reach out with your right hand and do the same spider-climb movement until you feel a stretch under your shoulder. Hold. Repeat on your left side.

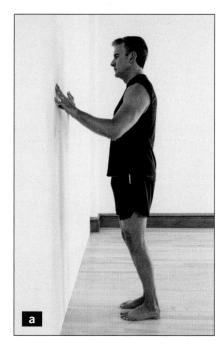
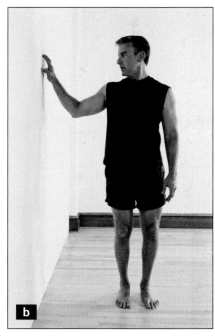

Shoulders >

Shoulder Twist

This exercise stretches the rotator cuff, a group of four muscles that stabilize the shoulder joint.

1. Stand straight with your feet hip-width apart and knees slightly bent, with arms hanging down by your side. Bend your elbows 90 degrees, keeping your upper arms next to your body so your forearms are parallel to the floor and pointed forward with thumbs pointing up (like shaking hands) **a**.

2. Keeping your thumbs up and elbows next to your body, move your hands away from each other until you feel a comfortable stretch in

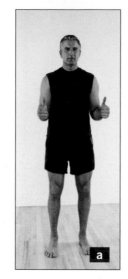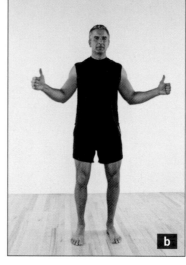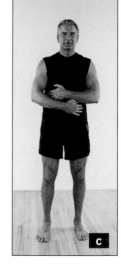

your shoulder **b**. Hold. Slowly bring your hands back toward you until the palms of your hands touch your body **c**. Hold.

TIP: On the return phase, to get palms to the front of your body, your hands will need to cross each other.

"Good Morning" Exercise

1. Stand straight with your feet hip-width apart and knees slightly bent, arms hanging down and hands on the front part of the opposite thigh.

2. Keeping your arms extended, lift your hands in a sideways and upward motion as high over your head as you can **a**. Hold for one second and return to the starting position. Do 6 repetitions.

TIP: Breathe in as you slowly lift your arms, and exhale as you return, which helps you establish a rhythm and trains you to breathe more deeply.

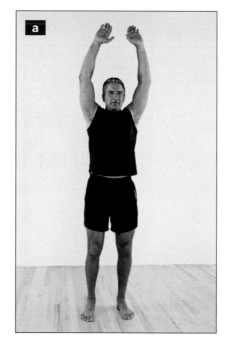

Scissors

This exercise stretches both the sides and backs of the shoulders.

1. Stand straight with your feet hip-width apart, arms by your side. With palms facing behind you, slowly swing your arms directly across the front of your body, with your right arm cutting in front of your left **a**.

2. Swing your arms back to the starting position, then cross them again, left arm cutting in front of the right. That is one repetition; do six.

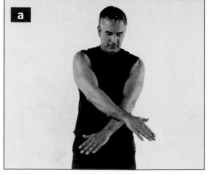

STRENGTH EXERCISES

`LEVEL 1`

Lying Lateral Raise

The flapping motion of this exercise provides a good all-around workout for muscles at the front, back, and sides of the shoulders. Helpful for people who struggle to comb or wash their hair.

1. Lie on the floor or your bed with your arms by your side close to your body.

2. Slowly and smoothly move your extended arms out to the side so they are at shoulder level **a**. Slowly return to the starting position.

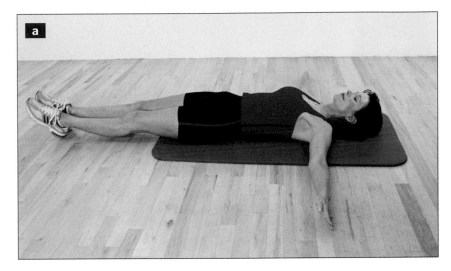

Lying Side Rotation

Here you work the shoulder's rotator cuff muscles as in the shoulder twist, but build strength by working against gravity.

1. Lie on the floor or a bed with legs extended and arms by your sides. Bend your elbows 90 degrees so that the tips of your fingers are facing the ceiling **a**.

2. Maintaining bent arms and keeping your elbows close to your body, slowly lower your hands to the sides as far as you comfortably can **b**. Slowly bring hands back to the starting position and beyond to touch the front of your body **c**.

NOTCH IT UP: To make this exercise more difficult, hold hand weights.

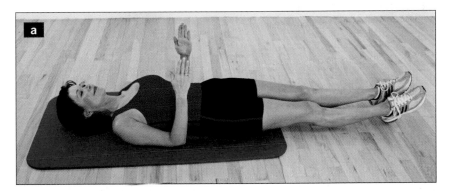

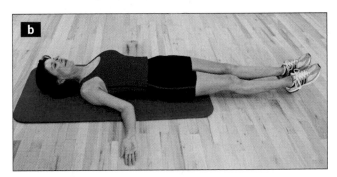

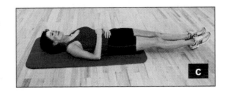

everyday *secrets*

Be consistent. Always start exercises on the same side of the body. Consistency makes keeping track of repetitions easier, especially when one repetition is completed only after both sides of the body have performed the movement.

Get a beat on pain. To make exercise more comfortable, try applying heat to painful joints or taking pain-relieving medications before you start. Be careful not to push yourself too hard during the workout. Analgesics can mask "good" pain that would otherwise tell you to hold back.

Play with balloons. Challenge your grandchildren to a balloon-batting contest. The team that keeps it off the ground longest gets the prize, but everybody is a winner because this is a terrific exercise for building strength and range of motion in all the muscles of the upper extremities from shoulders and arms to wrists and fingers.

continued on page 80

Modified Around the World

This exercise helps to build mobility, strength, and endurance for short over-the-head activities such as washing your hair.

1. Stand straight with your feet hip-width apart and knees slightly bent, arms hanging down and palms facing your thighs **a**. Slowly raise your extended arms out to the side until your hands reach the level of your shoulders **b**.

2. Keeping your arms at shoulder level, move your hands to the front and touch your thumbs together **c**. Slowly lower your arms in front of you until your palms touch the front of your thighs.

3. Do the entire exercise in reverse, raising hands to the front, moving them to the sides, and lowering them back to the starting position to complete one repetition.

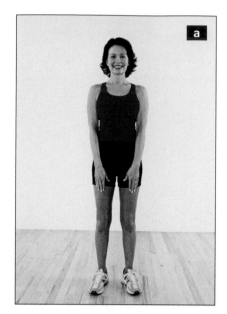

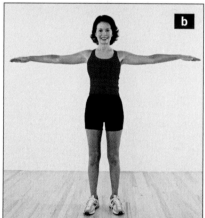

AT THE *Fitness Center*

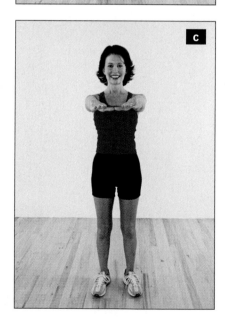

If you have access to good-quality exercise machines, here's what to use for your shoulders:

OVERHEAD PRESS
This exercise works like an overhead press using dumbbells, but guides your movement as you raise your arms against resistance.

LEVEL 2

Upright Row

Some people have trouble bending their elbows enough to do this exercise completely at first, but regular practice helps build range of motion not only in your shoulders, but your elbows as well.

1. Stand straight with your feet hip-width apart and knees slightly bent, arms hanging down and hands resting on the front of your thighs.

2. Keeping your hands close to your body, slowly bring your hands up your front so that your elbows move out to the side until they reach about the level of your shoulders, with your hands at the level of your chest 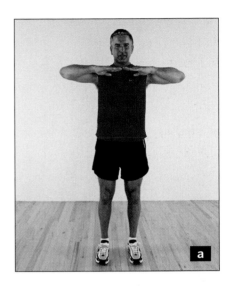. Hold for one second, then slowly lower your hands back to the starting position.

TIP: If it's difficult to raise your arms, just bring them to a level that feels comfortable.

NOTCH IT UP: To provide an extra challenge to muscles, hold a bit longer at the top of the lift. To significantly add resistance, hold hand weights.

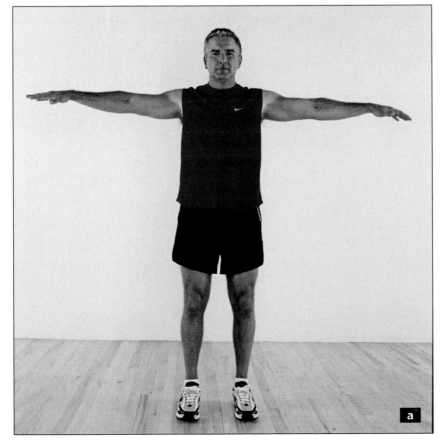

Standing Lateral Raise

This is the same basic movement as the lying lateral raises in level 1, but works more of the front, back, and sides of the shoulders because you're working against gravity.

1. Stand straight with your feet hip-width apart and knees slightly bent, arms hanging down by your side, palms facing your body.

2. Keeping your arms extended, smoothly raise your hands out to the side until they reach the level of your shoulders [a]. Slowly lower your hands to the starting position.

[73]

Front Raise

Varying the direction of the lift in this exercise concentrates resistance on the muscles at the front of your shoulders.

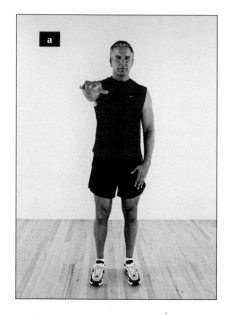

1. Stand straight with your feet hip-width apart and knees slightly bent, arms hanging down at the front of your thighs. Keeping your arms extended, slowly raise your right hand straight in front of you until it reaches the level of your shoulders **a**.

2. Slowly return to the starting position and repeat with the other arm to complete one repetition.

Around the World

This exercise works muscles surrounding the shoulder and helps develop coordinated movement. Similar to the modified around-the-world exercise in level 1, it requires you to lift your arms higher and extends your range of motion.

1. Stand straight with your feet hip-width apart and knees slightly bent, arms hanging down by your side and palms facing your thighs. Slowly raise your extended arms out to the side **a** until they go up over your head, turning your palms forward as you raise them so that your thumbs touch over your head **b** .

2. Slowly lower your extended arms in front of you until your palms touch the front of your thighs **c** . Reverse the move, raising your arms in front of you over your head, separating your hands and lowering your arms to the starting position to complete one repetition.

TIP: Make your movements smooth and fluid, not jerky, taking about three seconds to raise arms above your head, another three seconds to lower them to the front.

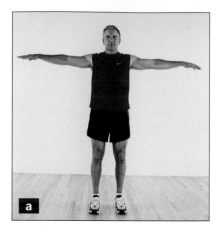

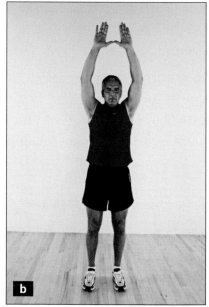

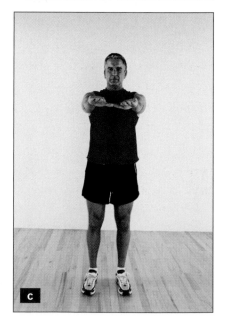

LEVEL 3

Weighted Lateral Raise

In a good example of how you can use the same basic exercise at three different levels of intensity, this move duplicates lateral raises in levels 1 and 2, but adds resistance with weights.

1. Stand straight with your feet hip-width apart and knees slightly bent, arms hanging down by your sides and a hand weight in each hand, palms facing your body.

2. Keeping your arms extended, slowly raise the weights out to the side until they reach the level of your shoulders **a**. Slowly lower the weights to the starting position.

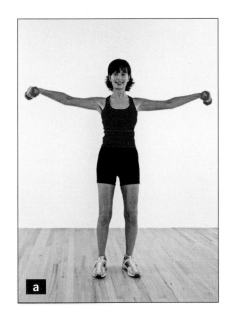

Overhead Dumbbell Press

Your shoulders get an excellent workout in this classic exercise—and so do the muscles of your upper back and the back of your arms.

1. Sit on a straight-backed chair or an exercise bench holding a hand weight in each hand. Keeping your elbows close to your body, bring the weights up to your shoulders **a**. This is your starting position.

2. Take a breath and slowly exhale as you push the weights over your head, turning your hands so your palms face forward. Lift your arms as far as you comfortably can, but don't lock your elbows **b**. Slowly lower the weights to the starting position, turning your hands palms-inward as they come down.

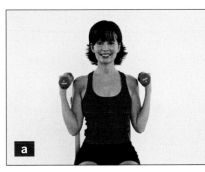

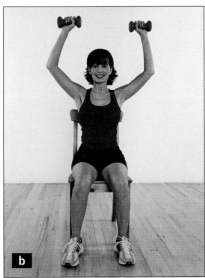

Weighted Front Raise

Again, the movement is the same as front raises in level 2, but weights add resistance and difficulty.

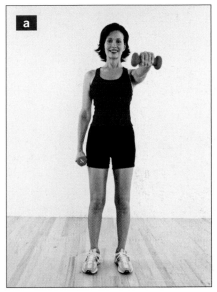

1. Stand straight with your feet hip-width apart and knees slightly bent. Grasp a hand weight in each hand, palms facing your body, arms hanging down at the front of your thighs. Keeping your arms extended, slowly raise the weight in your right hand straight in front of you until it reaches the level of your shoulders **a**.

2. Slowly return to the starting position and repeat with the left arm to complete one repetition.

TIP: To avoid straining your joints, don't lock your elbows, but consistently keep your arms slightly bent through the entire exercise.

At first glance, having strong abs seems more important for looking good on the beach than beating arthritis. But these large muscles are critical for support of the torso, and making them stronger contributes to improved posture—an important goal of physical activity for people with arthritis. Proper posture decreases stress throughout the body's joints, including those of the neck, spine, hips, knees, and ankles. When your muscles and bones are in proper alignment, joints work more efficiently, and you get better support from surrounding muscles, ligaments, and tendons.

STRETCHES

Seated Torso Twist

1. Sit in a straight-backed chair, preferably one with arms, with feet flat on the floor and legs bent 90 degrees **a** .

2. Turn your upper body at the waist to the right so that you're looking over your right shoulder **b** . Relax and hold, breathing normally. Come back to the starting position and repeat on the other side.

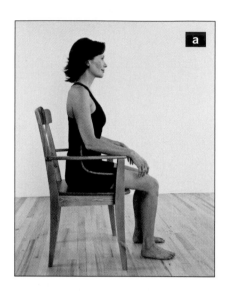

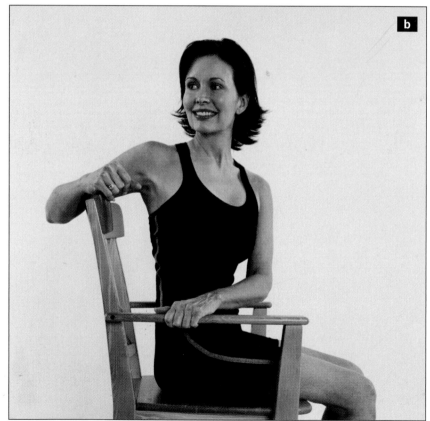

TIPS:
• To get an even better stretch, grab the arm of the chair to pull your body comfortably around using the hand on the side toward which you're twisting.

• If you're especially tight, do a second twist on each side after you finish your first complete set.

Ball Stretch

For this exercise, you'll need a fitness ball (scaled to your size) to provide a cushioned arch to your back that stretches the latticework of muscles throughout your abdomen.

1. Lie on your back with the ball positioned under your upper back, your hips lowered toward the floor, and your knees bent about 90 degrees **a**.

2. Slowly straighten your knees so that you roll on your back along the ball, keeping your feet on the floor and your hands over your stomach—or wherever they feel most comfortable—until you feel a stretch in your abdominal area **b**.

TIPS:
• If you feel you need greater stability, place your feet wider than shoulder-width apart.

• As you become more confident using the ball, try putting your arms over your head, which enhances the stretch and challenges your balance, providing a mild workout for leg muscles.

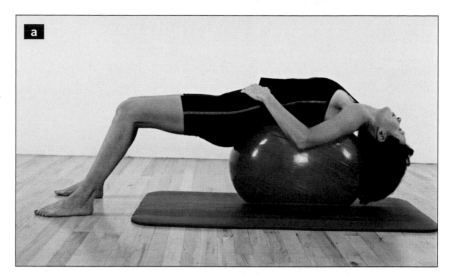

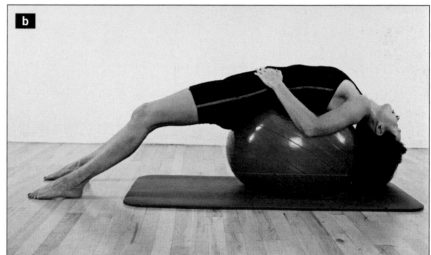

Lying Total Body Stretch

1. Lie on your back with your legs extended and feet together or about hip-width apart.

2. Extend your arms straight over your head and stretch your legs and toes, making your entire body as long as comfortably possible **a**. Hold.

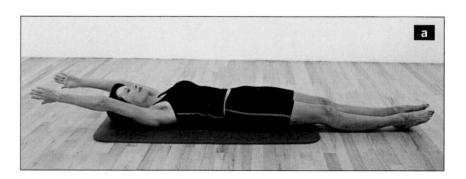

TIP: Take a deep breath before you begin the stretch, and exhale as you extend your hands and feet, then breathe normally as you hold, which enhances the stretch. Don't hold your breath, which prevents the abdominal muscles from relaxing.

STRENGTH EXERCISES

Modified Abdominal Curl

The curl is a fundamental part of any well-rounded routine, but the hand position on this version creates less resistance than in a standard curl.

1. Lie on your back with feet flat on the floor, knees bent, and your arms at your sides **a** .

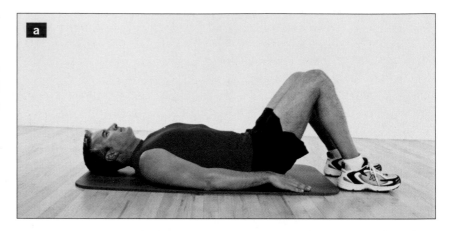

2. Raising your head, use your abdominal muscles to pull your shoulders off the floor so you can look at the top of your knees **b** . Keep enough space to fit a baseball between your chin and chest as you come up, and slide your hands forward along the floor as you move your shoulders off the floor.

3. Slowly lower your shoulders back to the floor.

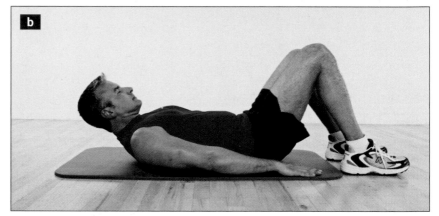

Basic Abdominal Curl

Start from the same position as in a modified curl (above), but with one difference: Put your hands across your chest, touching each hand to the opposite shoulder **a** . This provides more resistance for ab muscles to overcome **b** .

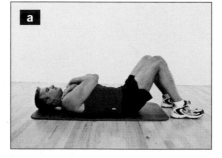
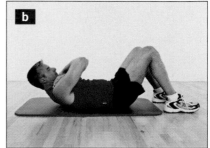

Basic Bicycle

This exercise is a favorite strength and endurance builder for athletes from diverse sports such as football, hockey, boxing, gymnastics, figure skating, and martial arts—yet it's easy to modify so that even people with chronic musculoskeletal problems can perform it.

1. Lie flat on your back with your legs straight and your hands behind or lightly touching your ears.

2. Lift your head off the floor and bring your left knee toward your head, stopping when your knee is about waist level and your thigh is perpendicular to the floor. At the same time, bring your right elbow toward the elevated knee so that your torso twists slightly and

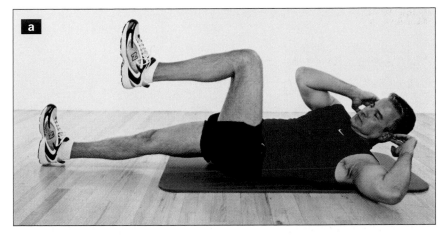

your elbow and knee are as close as possible over your abdomen 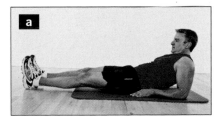.

3. Slowly return to the starting position. Rest for one second and repeat with the opposite limbs.

TIP: This exercise should take about 5 seconds, with 2 seconds to bring knee and elbow close, and 3 seconds to return. As you become stronger, reduce the resting time for a more difficult workout. All motions should be smooth and controlled, which keeps resistance on muscles longer and improves strength and tone more quickly.

Flutter Kick

This exercise helps build abdominal strength, but also enhances coordination if you swim.

1. Lie on your back, propped on your elbows, with your feet straight out in front of you, toes pointed toward the ceiling [a].

2. Lift your right heel 4 to 6 inches off the ground [b]. Bring it back to the floor, then lift and return the left leg in the same way to complete one repetition. Continue this kicking motion until you finish a set.

TIP: Though this move resembles swimming, don't kick fast like you're in the water, but keep movements slow and controlled, taking one second to lift and one second to return.

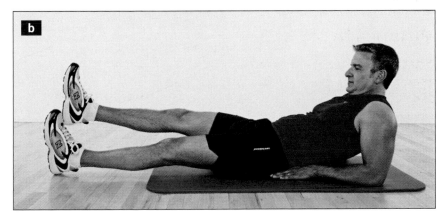

everyday *secrets*

Use the stairs. The familiar advice to take stairs instead of an elevator seems like a great way to build exercise into your day—if you don't work on the 14th floor. But don't think "all or nothing." You can walk up to the second floor, catch the elevator there, and ride the rest of the way. As you get stronger, take more flights and ride less.

Try two for one. Taking stairs two at a time doubles the exercise—you get the benefits of stair-climbing plus lunging. (And you may even beat the elevator.)

Walk, don't slouch. You can enhance the benefits of walking by practicing good posture as you stride. Hold your body so that shoulders and hips are aligned without arching your back. Keep your elbows close to your body. Let arms swing freely forward and back in a straight line.

continued on page 86

LEVEL 3

Advanced Abdominal Curl

Lift your head and shoulders off the floor just as you do with modified and basic curls, but in this version, touch your hands lightly behind your ears, which adds even greater resistance **a**.

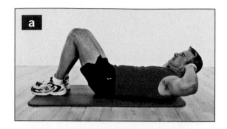

TIP: Don't hold your head in your hands to do curls. That tends to make you pull your head up with your hands, which puts pressure on the back of your upper spine. Instead, touch your hands lightly behind your ears **b**.

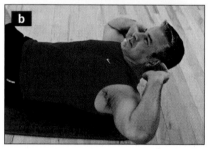

Advanced Flutter Kick

As with the flutter kick in level 2, you move your feet up and down as if swimming. In this exercise, however, you start with both feet one to two inches off the ground and keep them elevated through the entire exercise **a**. Take slightly less time to complete one kick, lifting in a half second, and returning in a half second (or whatever speed feels most comfortable) **b**.

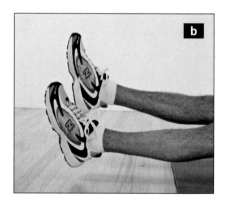

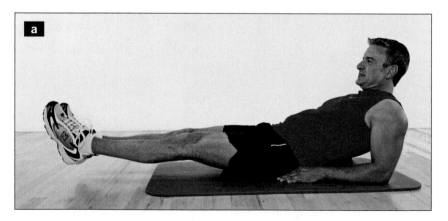

Advanced Bicycle

The movements with this exercise are the same as the basic bicycle in level 1. The difference:

With this advanced version, in the starting position, hold both your heels one to two inches off the floor, and keep both feet elevated through the entire exercise. At the same time, hold your head and shoulders off the floor 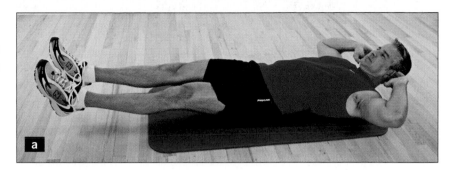. This constant resistance prevents rest between repetitions, making the advanced bicycle considerably more difficult than the basic version 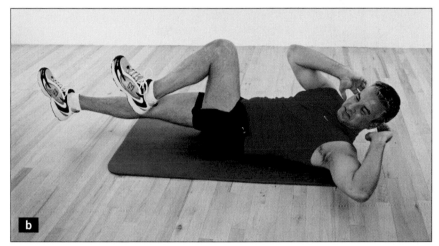.

Ball Curl

Consider this exercise a how-low-can-you-go challenge—but use an exercise ball instead of a limbo bar.

1. Sit up straight on the ball, crossing each hand across your chest to touch the opposite shoulder. Place feet flat on the floor, with your knees bent at about 90 degrees **a**.

2. Slowly lean backward while keeping the ball from rolling **b**. Lean back as far as you can while still maintaining balance. Slowly return to the starting position for one repetition.

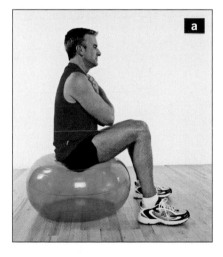

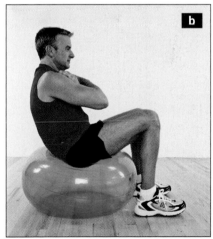

TIP: Don't worry about achieving a certain angle with your backward lean: The idea is to move as far as is comfortable—but if you consistently do the exercise, you'll make strides in both strength and balance that will allow you to lean back farther.

NOTCH IT UP: To make this exercise even more difficult, put your hands by your ears, which transfers weight to your upper body and increases resistance on your abdominal muscles.

Arthritis in the spine causes pain and stiffness, but can also lead to effects elsewhere in the body, such as weakness in the arms or legs. Getting up and walking is one of the most important ways to exercise the back, but you can also target the muscles that support the spine and help protect its joints. Even if you don't have arthritis in your spine, the torso-building exercises in this section can help prevent back pain—an exceedingly common condition—from making arthritis seem worse.

STRETCHES

Standing Posture Exercise

Your posture may suffer if arthritis has made you guard your movements by, for example, rounding your shoulders or leaning to one side. This exercise helps train your body to maintain proper alignment.

1. Stand with your back against a wall with your heels as close to the wall as possible.

2. Touch the wall with your shoulders and the back of your head 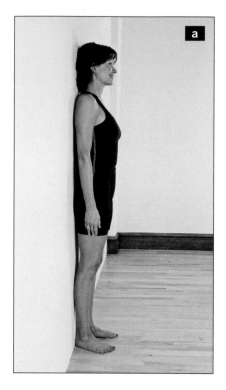. Register how your body feels in this good-posture position. Hold for 15 to 30 seconds—but try to carry yourself in this position as much as possible throughout your day.

Low Back Knees to Chest

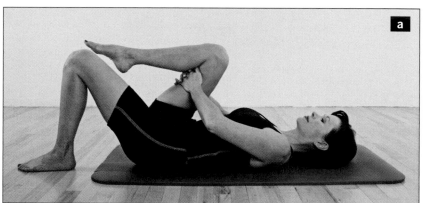

Though similar to the knees-to-chest exercise in the knees and hips section, this exercise keeps one foot flat on the floor, which bypasses the hip flexor muscles and provides a better stretch for the low back.

1. Lie on your back with your right leg fully extended and your left knee bent with the foot flat on the floor. Bring your right knee up to the level of your waist, keeping your left foot planted.

2. Put your hands in the crook of your leg behind your right thigh and gently pull your knee toward your right shoulder a. Stop when you feel a slight stretch. Hold and gently return to the starting position. Repeat on the other side.

Pelvic Twist

1. Lie on your back with your knees bent, feet flat on the floor, and arms extended straight out to your sides **a** .

2. Gently lower both knees to your right side until you feel a slight stretch in your left lower back and hip area **b** . Hold and return to the starting position. Repeat on the other side.

TIP: To get the most from this stretch, keep both shoulders on the floor.

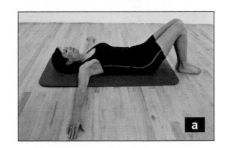

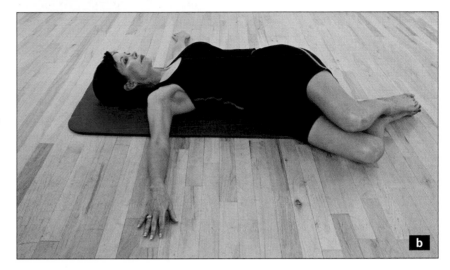

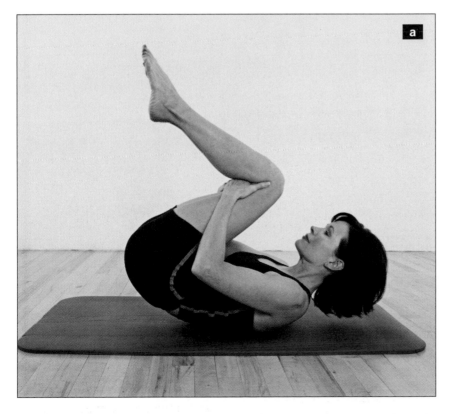

Rocking Chair

The rocking motion of this stretch helps develop muscle control and, by contracting the stomach muscles, automatically causes the nervous system to relax back muscles, allowing a better stretch.

1. Lie on your back with knees bent and feet flat on the floor. Reach up and put your hands behind your knees.

2. Pull both knees toward your shoulders. When you feel a slight stretch in your low back and buttocks, gently rock back and forth on your rounded back **a** .

TIP: This exercise is most comfortable when done on a rug, exercise mat, or bed.

Cat Stretch

This is a classic back stretch, often used in yoga routines.

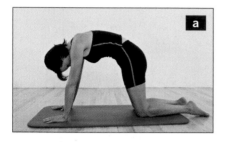

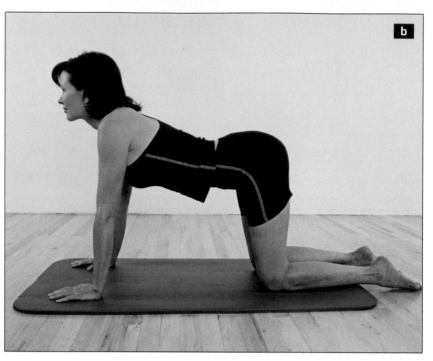

1. Get on your hands and knees. Tuck your chin toward your chest and tighten your stomach muscles to arch your back **a** . Hold.

2. Relax, raising your head so you're looking straight ahead while pushing your stomach toward the floor **b** . Hold.

Cross-Legged Seated Stretch

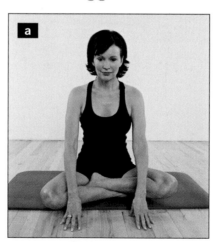

1. Sit on the floor with your legs crossed and hands in front of you **a** . Lean forward gently with your head down, rounding your back and "walking" your fingers forward until you feel a stretch in your lower and middle back **b** . Hold.

2. Walk your hands back to your legs and return to the starting position.

TIP: For a balanced stretch to both sides of the back, do this exercise twice, switching the leg that is crossed over the top.

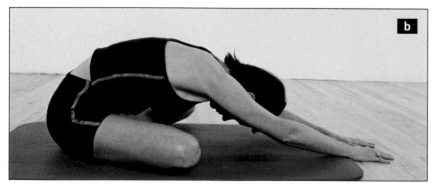

Seated Body Hang

If you feel light-headed when you lean over, skip this stretch.

1. Sit in a straight-backed chair (with or without arms), with your feet flat on the floor and your hands on your knees **a**.

2. Gently lean forward, moving your hands toward the floor between your feet until you feel a stretch in your middle and lower back **b**. Hold.

TIP: To return to the starting position if you have back pain, put your hands or forearms on your knees and push yourself up.

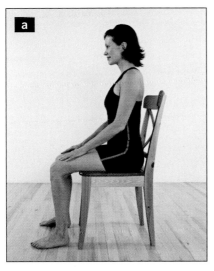

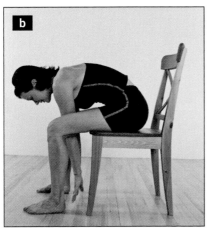

Side Bend and Twist

In the second part of this move, raising your hands helps keep your head in proper alignment with your upper body.

1. Stand straight with your feet about hip-width apart, arms at your sides.

2. Gently lean to the right, sliding your hand down the side of your thigh toward your knee until you feel a slight stretch on the left side of your waist **a**. Hold. Return to the starting position and repeat on the other side.

3. Return to the starting position and bend your elbows at about 90 degrees so that your hands are in front of you. Rotate your upper body so that your hands move to the right side while keeping your hips pointed straight ahead until you feel a stretch in your left lower back **b**. Hold.

4. Slowly return to the starting position and repeat on the other side.

TIP: If you feel unbalanced during the side bend, place your feet farther apart for greater stability, or try a similar move from a sitting position.

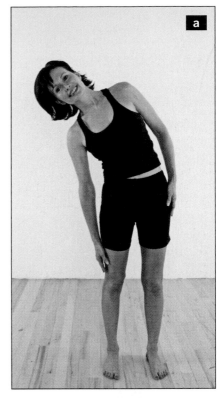

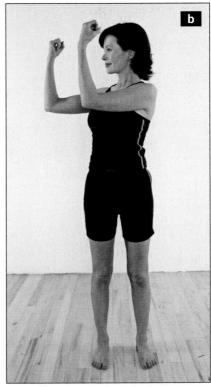

continued on page 93

STRENGTH EXERCISES

LEVEL 1

Lying Alternating Arm Raise

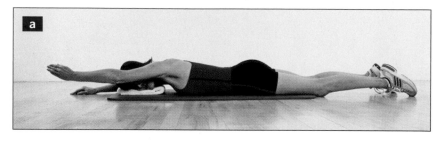

This exercise focuses on the muscles of the neck, upper back, and shoulder blade area.

1. Lie on your stomach with your legs extended, your head straight down on a pillow or folded towel or turned to the side, whichever is more comfortable, and your arms extended directly in front of you.

2. Smoothly raise your left arm as far as comfortably possible **a**. Hold one second and lower. Repeat with the other arm to complete one repetition.

Lower-Body Extension

This exercise is not only excellent for the hips (you'll find it in that section as well), but also works the muscles of the lower back.

1. Get down on your hands and knees on the floor, a rug, or an exercise mat.

2. Extend your left leg out behind you, keeping your foot about one inch off the floor as you straighten your knee **a**. Return to the starting position and repeat with the other leg to complete one repetition.

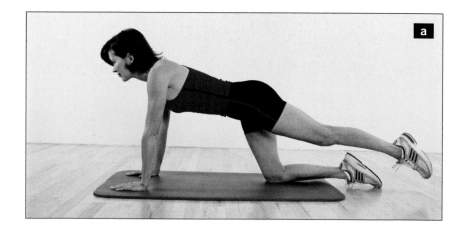

LEVEL 2

Superman

This exercise hits muscles throughout the spine from the base of your head to the buttocks, all of which add stability to your spine.

1. Lie on your stomach with your arms extended directly in front of you, your legs straight out behind you, and your eyes looking at your hands **a**.

2. Holding your chin off the floor, gently lift both arms and both feet about one inch, hold one second and lower to the floor for one repetition **b** .

TIP: If you feel discomfort in the back of your neck, keep your eyes facing the floor and rest your head on a pillow instead of lifting your chin off the floor.

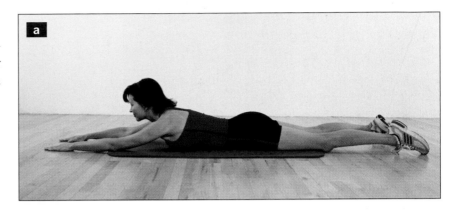

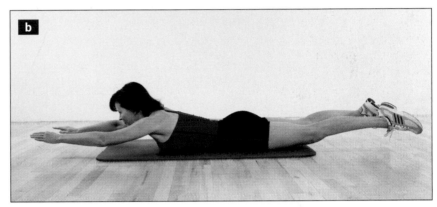

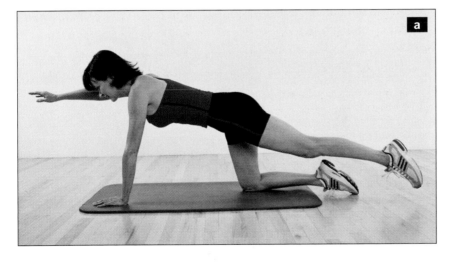

Bird Dog

As with the lower-body extension, this exercise works muscles in both the back and hips, so it's an excellent choice for either area (see also Knees and Hips, page 62).

1. Get down on your hands and knees on the floor, a rug, or an exercise mat.

2. Extend your left leg out behind you, keeping your foot about one inch off the floor as you straighten your knee. At the same time you extend your left leg, reach out straight in front of you with your right arm **a**.

3. Return to the starting position and repeat with the other leg and arm to complete one repetition.

[87]

Bent Single Arm Row

This exercise is best done on an exercise bench, but can also be performed using a sturdy armless chair.

1. Stand by the front corner of an armless chair with your feet about hip-width apart, holding a hand weight in your right hand.

2. Bend over and place your left hand on the chair so that your back is parallel with the floor. Lower the weight so your right arm is straight **a**.

3. Lift the weight toward your chest, holding your elbow close to your body and moving it straight up toward the ceiling. Stop when the weight is just below chest level

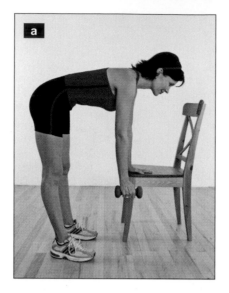

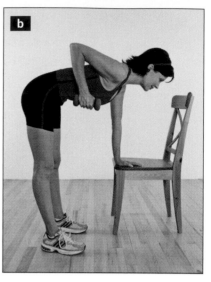

b. Hold for one second and slowly lower the weight to the straight-arm starting position. After completing a set, repeat with the other arm.

TIP: If you have pain or discomfort in the hand or wrist you lean on, instead rest your elbow and forearm on the back of the chair for support.

LEVEL 3

Dead Lift

If your function level is good and you perform the movement correctly, this exercise will strengthen your lower back and build better posture.

1. Stand with your feet about hip-width apart, knees slightly bent **a**.

2. Keeping knees slightly flexed, bend over at the waist and lower your hands straight down toward your feet, keeping your hands close to your legs at first, then moving them out to your toes **b**. Return to the standing position for one repetition.

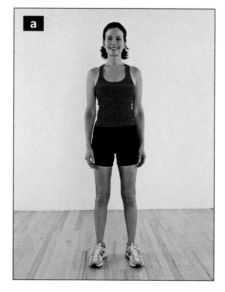

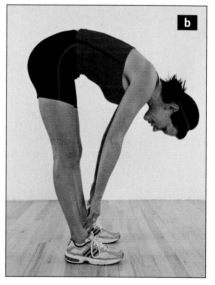

TIPS:
• Avoid this exercise if you have back problems or low back pain.
• If you lack flexibility in hamstrings and hips, start by bending so hands go only to knee. Don't lock your knees.

NOTCH IT UP: You make this exercise more difficult—and more worthy of caution—by using hand weights. Attempt this only after you've developed strength and flexibility in your lower back by doing the exercise without weights.

Advanced Bird Dog

Building on the basic bird dog move in level 2, this more advanced exercise not only works muscles of the hips, but also the back and shoulders.

1. Get down on your hands and knees on the floor, a rug, or an exercise mat.

2. Extend your left leg out behind you, raising your foot so that your entire leg is parallel to the floor—a more strenuous position than in the basic bird dog. At the same time, reach out straight in front of you with your right arm **a** .

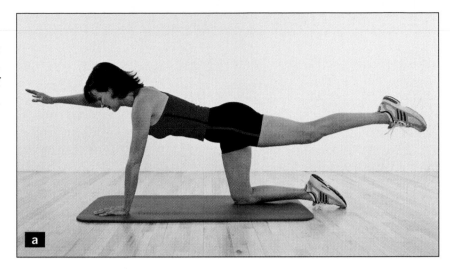

3. Return to the starting position and repeat with the other leg and arm to complete one repetition. Continue alternating legs and arms until you finish a set.

AT THE *Fitness Center*

If you have access to good-quality exercise machines, here's what to use for your back and spine:

SEATED ROW MACHINE
For best results, if you have a choice of handle grips, select one in which the handles are vertical; if there are multiple grip positions, choose the innermost one.

PULL-DOWN MACHINE
You may see other exercisers pulling the bar behind their heads, but it's best to avoid such a move, which puts excess stress on the shoulder joint. Do the exercise in a slow and controlled manner, keeping your back straight so you don't use any momentum to pull the bar down. To make this exercise more difficult, place your hands closer to the ends of the bar. For another variation, rotate your palms to face inward (as if doing a chin-up), and position your hands 2 to 3 inches apart, which works muscles lower down the sides of your back.

Chest muscles play a vital role in stabilizing the multidirectional shoulder joints, which are essential to a wide variety of every-day tasks, such as carrying heavy loads and opening doors. Building strong chest muscles also helps improve posture, taking pressure off the spine. What's more, many exer-cises for chest muscles also work the hands and arms, conditioning muscles from all of these areas to work together.

STRETCHES

Seated Chest Stretch

This stretch for the upper chest and front shoulders can be done from either a standing or sitting position.

1. Place your hands at the back of your head with fingers interlocked **a**.

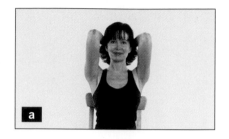

2. Gently move your elbows back-ward or behind you until you feel a stretch at the front of your shoul-ders and the top of your chest **b**.

TIP: If you find you're especially stiff in this area, assume the starting position in a straight-backed chair and have a part-ner assist by gently pulling your elbows back from behind the chair. As soon as you feel a slight stretch in your chest, tell your partner to stop pulling. Or do the stretch lying on your back with knees bent and both feet flat on the floor.

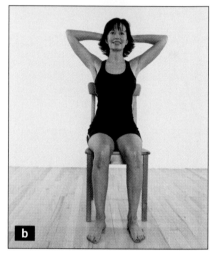

Lying Total Body Stretch

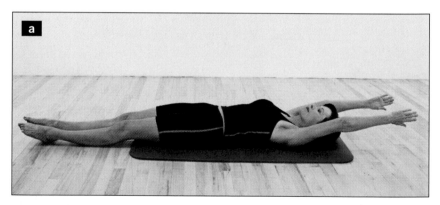

By putting your hands over your head, this stretch (a double-duty move also described in the abdom-inal section, page 77) lengthens chest muscles in a different direc-tion than the other stretches.

1. Lie on your back on a bed or a mat with your legs extended and

feet together or comfortably apart at about hip width.

2. Extend your arms straight over your head and stretch your legs and toes, making your entire body as long as comfortably possible **a**. Hold.

Wall Stretch

1. Start by standing with your right side next to a wall, then take one regular-size step forward with your left foot. Place your right forearm vertically against the wall, with your elbow bent at 90 degrees so that your upper arm is parallel to the floor and your hand is pointing toward the ceiling.

2. Keeping your back heel flat on the floor, slowly bend your front knee so that your body moves forward and you feel a stretch in your chest and upper arm **a**. Hold and repeat on the other side.

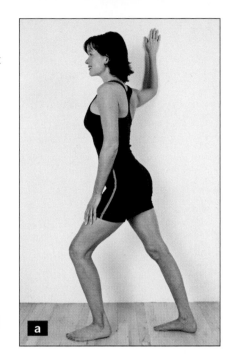

STRENGTH EXERCISES

LEVEL 1

Wall Push-Up

1. From a standing position about 12 to 18 inches from a wall, put your hands on the wall about shoulder-width apart at chest level, with palms flat and fingers pointed toward the ceiling **a**.

2. Slowly lower your chin toward the wall **b**. Smoothly push back from the wall to the starting position.

TIP: As you lower yourself to the wall, keep elbows out to the side. That works the chest muscles better than keeping elbows close to the body, which shifts the load more to the triceps muscles of the arms. If you feel pain in your hands or wrist, try placing hands farther apart or closer together on the wall, which may prove more comfortable. If not, you may want to choose another exercise.

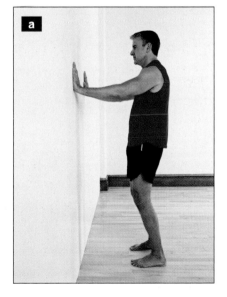

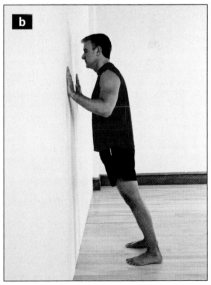

Chest Fly

This is a weightlifting move without the weight. But if you're not already strength training, this exercise can make you stronger without causing soreness from working against too much resistance.

1. Lie on the floor with knees bent and feet flat. Extend your hands toward the ceiling with your arms slightly bent, palms facing each other 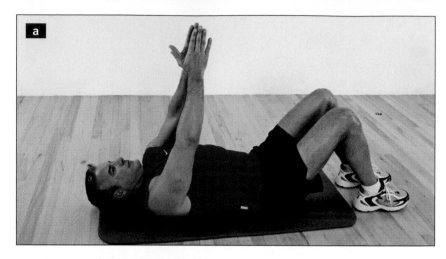.

2. Slowly inhale as you lower your extended arms until your hands are just above the floor **b** . Hold for one second and, exhaling, raise your extended arms and bring your hands together at the starting position.

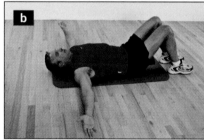

TIP: Keep your elbows slightly bent through the entire movement, not changing the angle, which would alter the amount of resistance on the muscles of the chest. This exercise can also be done lying on a bed.

LEVEL 2

Weighted Chest Fly

This exercise follows the same basic motion as the chest fly in level 1, but adds hand weights for greater resistance. While this is best done on an exercise bench, a floor mat will do.

1. Place your hand weights in a convenient location on either side of a floor mat, then lie down on your back with knees bent and feet flat to the floor, shoulder-width apart. Carefully grab your hand weights and press them toward the ceiling, holding them with palms facing each other **a** . This is your starting position.

2. Maintaining a slight bend in your elbow, inhale as you smoothly lower the weights to your sides until your upper arm is nearly parallel to the

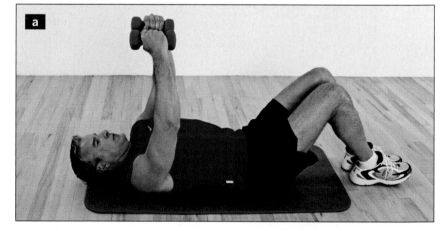

floor **b** . Try not to put the weights on the floor, but rather hold them a few inches above. Exhale as you pull your hands back up toward the starting position.

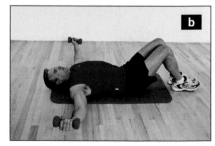

TIP: Keep your lifting movement smooth and controlled to cut momentum and prevent the weights from knocking against each other at the top of the lift.

LEVEL 3

Ball Push-Up

This exercise is even more challenging than a traditional push-up (which you could use as a level 2 exercise) because you need to draw on stabilizing muscles to keep the ball from rolling from side to side.

1. Put the fitness ball against a wall and place your hands on the top of the ball about shoulder-width apart, with your arms straight, your legs extended and your feet about hip-width apart.

2. Inhaling, slowly lower yourself until your chest touches the ball **a**. Exhaling, push your body away from the ball to the starting position.

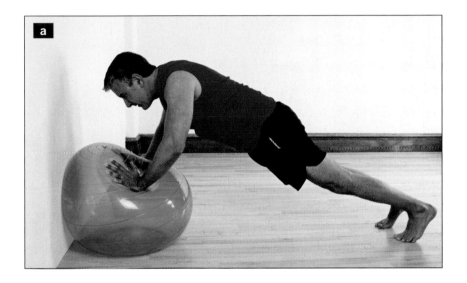

AT THE *Fitness Center*

If you have access to good-quality exercise machines, here's what to use for your chest:

CHEST PRESS MACHINE

Keep your elbows aligned with your hands through the entire exercise to avoid putting excessive pressure on the hand joints. When grabbing hold, make sure the bar is pressing on the pad of your palm. If the bar isn't padded and you find it uncomfortable, try placing a sponge or towel in your hand as you grip the bar for added cushioning—but be careful this doesn't compromise your grip. Doing one set places this exercise at level 2; adding sets as you get stronger notches it up to level 3.

everyday
secrets

Break it up. Sitting still—hunched over a desk or a computer station, for example—can cause tension and strain that makes muscles and joints more painful. To avoid this discomfort, take a short break at least every 10 minutes or so (set a timer if you're really concentrating). Stand up and walk around for a minute; it relieves tension (especially in the back) and mildly exercises stiff muscles and joints.

Make breaks automatic. While working at your desk, stash items that you use occasionally (but not constantly) beyond your reach. That way, you'll be forced to get up every now and then—in effect, taking a break and mildly exercising without feeling like you've stopped working.

Play ball. Just because it's fitness equipment doesn't mean you can't have fun with an exercise ball. Example: Making a lunge to bounce a ball against a wall with your hands provides a workout for wrist, hands, shoulders, chest, back, hips, and knees.

continued on page 96

Your neck muscles are probably fairly strong already because they're accustomed to handling an ample amount of resistance: the weight of your head. But that's not all neck muscles do. They also help maintain proper posture, which relieves stress on the overall structure of the neck and spine, and are critical for daily functions such as looking over your shoulder when backing out of a parking space. Daily demands go a long way toward keeping neck muscles in shape. Yet in some cases, constant muscular tension in the neck can contribute to headaches and back pain, especially if arthritis makes you limit your head movement. Your goal, then, isn't to progressively build strength, but to improve flexibility, tone, and endurance. That's why the exercises in this section can be done at all three function levels.

To progress, simply add repetitions as you become stronger and more comfortable.

STRETCHES

Neck Side Bend

1. Sit up straight in a chair with your eyes looking directly ahead **a** .

2. Slowly lower your right ear toward your right shoulder, stopping when you feel a slight stretch in the muscles on the left side of your neck **b** . Hold. Return to the starting position and repeat on the other side.

TIP: The weight of your head is sufficient to produce a good stretch for functional (but not excessive) range of motion—so there's no need to pull the side of your head down with your hand. You can do a similar stretch for muscles at the back of your neck by slowly letting your head dip forward. However, avoid stretching your neck by leaning your head back: This position can interfere with blood supply to the brain and may cause faintness.

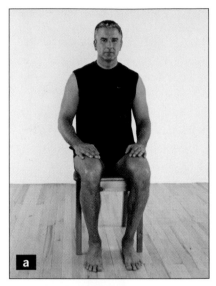

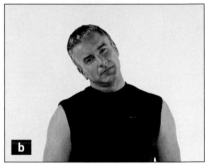

Neck Turn

You can do this exercise anytime, anywhere, while sitting or standing. But if your neck is sensitive or in pain, do this exercise lying down to lessen the pressure.

1. Sit or stand up straight with your eyes looking directly ahead.

2. Slowly and smoothly move your head to the right side until you feel a slight stretch in the muscles on the opposite side of your neck **a** . Relax and hold. Slowly return to the starting position and repeat on the other side.

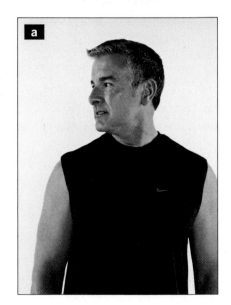

Posture Stretch

You might think this doesn't qualify as a stretching exercise—there's virtually no physical effort involved. Still, this visualizing exercise has excellent posture-building benefits.

1. While standing with feet about hip-width apart, imagine that there's a string attached to the top of your head pulling you up and making you an inch taller, and adjust your body accordingly **a**. This will help you understand what it feels like to sit up straight, eliminate rounding of the shoulders, and

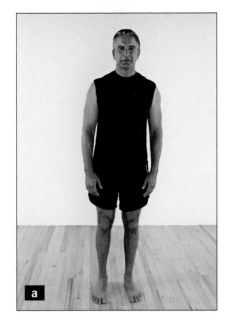

align your head and neck. Practicing this mind/body exercise continuously will automatically improve your posture and make your entire body fall into better alignment, easing muscle tension and helping to relieve pain.

TIP: Don't push up with your toes when doing this exercise standing: The goal is to *feel* like you're being pulled up an inch; you don't actually need to be taller. If you have trouble standing straight or have pain in the hips or knees, perform this exercise sitting in a chair.

STRENGTH EXERCISES

"Yes" Exercise

This isometric exercise can be done almost anywhere.

1. Sit in a chair with your back against the chair and your neck slightly bent forward as if you're nodding yes **a**.

2. Press your head forward while applying gentle resistance to your forehead with either a pillow or your palms **b**. Hold as follows, according to your function level:

• 3 seconds for level 1
• 6 seconds for level 2
• 10 seconds for level 3

Relax and repeat one more time.

3. Press your head backward while applying gentle resistance by placing both hands behind your head with fingers interlaced **c**.

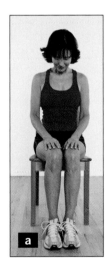
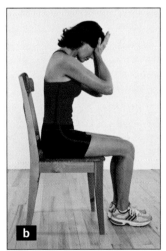
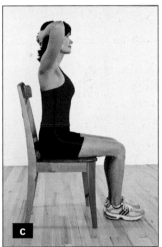

TIP: For a variation on the pressing-forward phase, get a similar effect using gravity by lying on your back and lifting your head an inch or two off the floor— as if you're doing an abdominal curl, but

without raising your shoulders off the floor. The pressing-back phase of this exercise looks relaxing, but it shouldn't be. Actively push your head back against your hands.

STR

Use good phone technique.
One of the most common causes of tension in the cervical spine is sloppy use of the telephone. It's not enough to stop cradling the handset between your ear and shoulder. You should also avoid holding it on just one side of your head— switch hands (and ears) regularly during a conversation. If you have a cell phone, use the hands-free earpiece/microphone that's included with it. Otherwise, pick up one at an electronics store.

Create a pain-free desk. Rearrange your desk to eliminate sources of strain on muscles and joints. Keep the objects you use often in a semicircle within arm's reach. When you grab something, bring it close to your body to use. Heavy objects such as reference books should be on your desk or a middle shelf nearby. Avoid reaching for objects over your head or behind you, especially if they're heavy. Stand up to get them.

continued on page 102

Resisted Side Press

Think of this as a side-to-side version of the "yes" exercise.

1. Sit up straight in a chair with your eyes focused forward and your head cocked slightly to the right.

2. Press your head toward your right shoulder while applying gentle resistance with the heel of your right hand against the side of your head above the ear **a**. Relax and repeat on the other side.

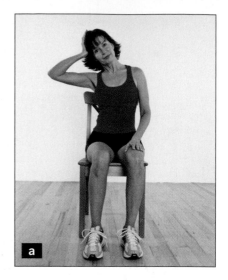

MASSAGES

Side Stroke

1. Place the fingers of your left hand on the right side of your neck just below your ear, and stroke muscles in a downward motion toward your collarbone **a**.

2. Lift your fingers and return to the starting position. Do three strokes and repeat on the other side.

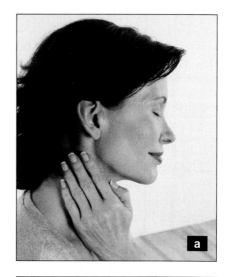

Vertebrae Press

1. Place your left hand on the back of your neck with fingers positioned on the right side of the neck bones just below the hairline.

2. Press with your fingers as you move your hand along the cervical spine from the base of your head to your shoulder **a**. Do this three times and repeat on the other side.

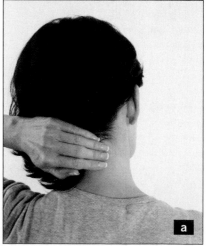

9 Ways to Prevent Stressed Muscles

For many people, the stresses of life—be they mental or physical—show up quickly in the neck muscles. Stretches and exercises can relieve a neck ache, but here are nine ways to avoid having your body tense up in the first place. And all are particularly good for arthritis as well!

1. Be like a cat and stretch often—and luxuriously. Your body wants to stretch, and often does so unconsciously. Stretching loosens the muscles, helps your blood flow, relieves your bones and joints, and refreshes your spirit. For a person with arthritis, stretching is as healthy a habit as you can develop. It can be a formal, multi-step routine, or it can be just standing up and exalting the sky.

2. Find more reasons to laugh. The obvious reason is that humor relieves the tensions of everyday life. But not so obvious are the physiological effects of a good laugh. Feel-good brain chemicals called endorphins are released when you laugh that ease pain and improve attitude. Plus, laughter stimulates the heart, lungs, muscles, and immune system.

3. Chop your to-do list in half. We know we're not going to get everything done that we want to in a day. And yet so many of us wake up with a set of expectations for the day that are grand beyond reason. Be fair to yourself: Make your task list reasonable, and achieve it. There's no better way to reduce physical and emotional stress than regularly feeling like a success.

4. Glory in hot water. The water soothes and supports the joints. The heat brings blood to your joints, muscles, and skin, flushing you with nutrients and relief. And the calmness of a soak in a tub or Jacuzzi makes life just seem better. Ask your doctor first if a Jacuzzi habit is healthy for you—the heat can alter your circulation.

5. Invest in your bed (and your bedding). There are pillows, and then there are pillows. Same for mattresses, mattress pads, sheets, and comforters. A bed that is firm but luxurious, that makes you say "ahhhh" when you lie down, that gives you the comfort you need for a great night's sleep, is a wonderful investment for your health and your joints.

6. Create a midday ritual. Perhaps it's a cup of tea, a walk, a stretch, a music break, or just a phone call. Whatever it is, take 5 to 15 minutes each afternoon for a personal break. Getting out of the intensity of everyday life for a short while is beneficial, both physically and emotionally. And by making it a constant ritual, you relax yourself merely by the knowledge that it is soon arriving.

7. Trust us: A good massage is one of life's greatest pleasures. Every month or so, skip the weekend trip to the hair salon and spend the money instead on a massage. The muscle and joint relief will be substantial.

8. Live your life in ebbs and flows. In exploring the optimal workouts for athletes, researchers are beginning to believe that the best training method is to exert for a short period and then rest, rather than doing prolonged periods of exertion. It's a theory that is applicable to all of us, particularly those with arthritis. Walk a few minutes; then relax a while. Clean for 15 minutes; then take a break. This way, you don't overtax muscles, and you give all the parts of your body a chance to recover before exerting again.

9. Let it be. If you are a human being, then certain truths are inevitable: The government is wrong; half your relatives are crazy; there's never enough money; work is unfair; you're surrounded by crazy drivers. You have a choice: Let it get to you, or don't let it get to you. Our recommendation: When a cause for anger dangles in front of you, don't take the bait. Life's too short to be angry all the time. And it's not fair to your body.

The muscles of the ankles and feet are small. You can give them a good workout using simple exercises with only small amounts of resistance. These exercises use body weight rather than special equipment. But the size of muscles isn't a measure of their importance: The muscles that support the ankle and foot joints are critical to your mobility in walking and climbing stairs. Body-weight exercises are ideal because they train the muscles in the ways you actually use them in daily life.

STRETCHES

Stair Calf Stretch

1. Stand on a stair with feet about hip-width apart, with your weight on the balls of your feet and your heels sticking over the edge of the stair **a**.

2. Slowly lower your heels until you feel a stretch in your calves and the backs of your ankles **b**. Hold and return to the starting position.

TIP: Hold on to the stair rail or wall to steady yourself and maintain control during the stretch. Because your entire body weight factors into this stretch, be careful not to drop your heels too far or too fast—and be sure to stretch both legs at once.

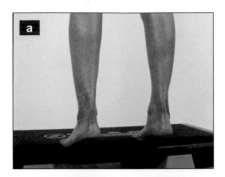

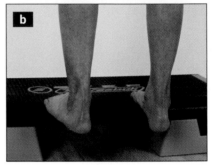

Ankle Circle

This is not a static stretch, but a range-of-motion exercise that promotes ankle mobility.

1. Sit in a chair with legs extended slightly so that heels rest on the floor about hip-width apart and toes point up at about a 45-degree angle.

2. Rotate from your ankles in a clockwise direction so that your toes trace circles in the air **a**. Do this 6 to 8 times.

3. Change direction, making counterclockwise circles.

TIPS:
• If you're comfortable making small circles, expand your range of motion by pushing or pulling toes as far in each direction as you can. Your feet don't have to touch. For example, you could do this exercise with feet dangling as you sit on the edge of your bed.

• To add a simultaneous resistance exercise for your legs, elevate your feet while performing the ankle motion.

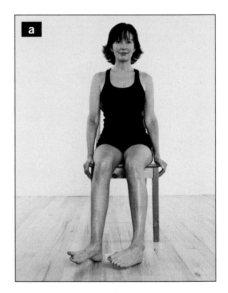

Runner's Calf Stretch

Always a popular way for runners to limber up their calves, this stretch is ideal for anyone who could use more lower-leg flexibility.

1. Stand with toes of both feet about 12 to 18 inches from a wall.

2. Supporting yourself against the wall with one or both hands, take a big step back with your right foot, keeping your left foot in place.

Bending your left knee, keep your right leg straight with your heel flat on the ground to produce a gentle tug at the back of your lower leg (Achilles tendon) **a**. Hold and return to the starting position. Repeat on the other side.

TIP: Move your hips forward to increase the stretch.

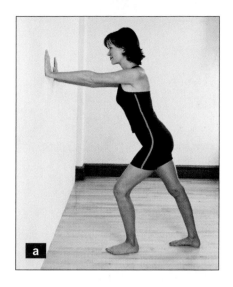

Seated Swivel

These moves give a more concentrated range-of-motion stretch to some of the muscles targeted by ankle circles, particularly those at the front and sides of your ankles.

1. Sit on the edge of a chair with feet flat on the floor about three to four inches apart.

2. Push up with your toes so that your heels rise off the floor. Turn your heels slowly and smoothly as far to the right as you comfortably can **a**. Hold.

3. Now turn heels slowly and smoothly to the left as far as you comfortably can **b**. Hold. Do this in both directions 6 to 8 times and return to the starting position.

4. Next, pull up with your toes so that they rise off the floor. Similar to the moves above, turn toes slowly and smoothly to the left and hold, then turn toes to the right and hold. Repeat 6 to 8 times.

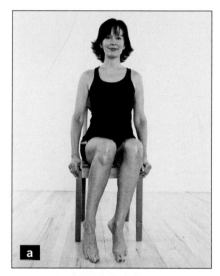

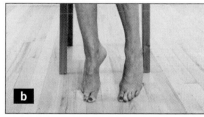

TIP: You may tend to swing your knees with the movement of this exercise, which is fine if it makes the motion more comfortable. As a rule, however, you'll get a better stretch if you keep your knees as steady as possible.

Toe Stretch and Curl

While sitting or standing, take your shoes off and simply stretch your toes apart as far as possible **a**. Try to wiggle your toes in as many directions as you can.

From a sitting or standing position with your shoes off, curl your toes as if you were trying to use your feet to grasp an object. Better yet, place a towel under your feet and repeatedly curl your toes to pull the towel closer **b**.

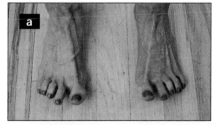

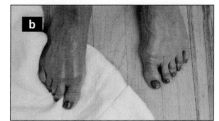

STRENGTH EXERCISES

Heel Raise

This exercise strengthens two major muscles in the calf and shores up the Achilles tendon.

1. Stand with your feet about hip-width apart, using a chair or wall to keep your balance.

2. Raise yourself on the balls of both feet so your heels lift off the floor as high as they comfortably can **a**. Slowly lower back to the floor.

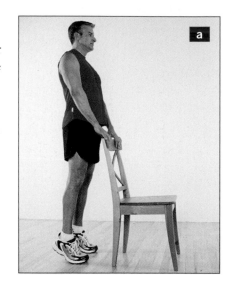

LEVEL 2

Stair Heel Raise

This exercise combines moves from the basic heel raises in level 1 and the stair calf stretches to work your calf and ankle muscles through a fuller (and more difficult) range of motion.

1. Stand on a stair with feet about hip-width apart, with your weight on the balls of your feet and your heels protruding over the edge of the stair.

2. Slowly lower your heels until you feel a stretch in your calves and the backs of your ankles **a**.

3. Lift your heels and stand as high on the balls of your feet as you comfortably can **b**. Hold for one second, then slowly lower to the starting position and repeat.

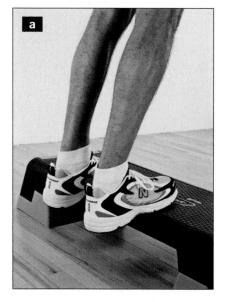
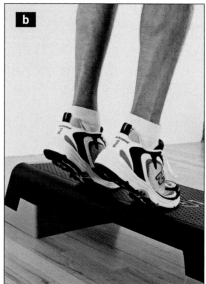

TIP: As with the stair calf stretch, be sure you stay under control through the entire motion, using a stair rail for support: Dropping heels suddenly below the level of the stair can overstretch the calves and strain the Achilles tendon.

Heel/Toe Raise

By combining two motions, this exercise works both the calves (when you're on the balls of your feet) and the muscles at the front of your shins (when you're on your heels).

1. Stand with both feet on the floor about hip-width apart using a chair, counter, or wall for balance.

2. Rise up on the balls of your feet so that your heels come off the floor as far as comfortably possible 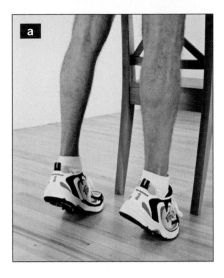. Hold for one second and slowly lower your heels to the floor (the starting position).

3. Elevate your toes and the front of your feet off floor as far as comfortably possible 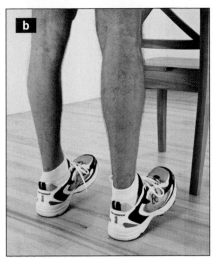. Hold for one second, then lower to floor to complete one repetition.

Ankle Roll

Doing this exercise may make you aware of muscles you didn't know you had—on the inside and outside of your ankles.

1. Sit in a chair with your feet flat on the floor about hip-width apart.

2. Using the muscles on the inside of your ankles, roll your feet outward along their outside edge so that the bottoms of your feet face toward each other 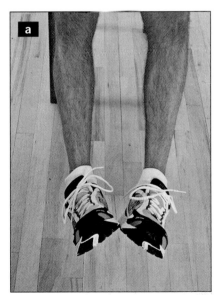. Keeping your ankles moving, return to the starting position.

3. Using the muscles on the outside of your ankles, roll your feet along their inside edge so that the bottoms of your feet face away from each other 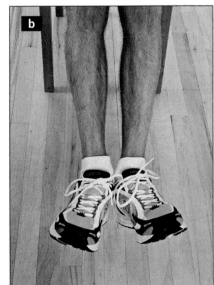.

TIP: Concentrate on your ankle muscles as you do the exercise. These muscles should be producing the movement in your feet, not your knees or legs.

continued on page 108

everyday *secrets*

Get the right angle. Tilting your head back to view a computer screen is a common source of neck tension, especially for people with bifocals. Instead, adjust the screen to eye level or slightly below eye level. If you can't make the screen lower, raise the height of your chair.

Keep wrists straight. To keep keyboard typing from aggravating wrist pain, don't let your wrists tilt upward to reach the keys. Keep hands and forearms in a straight line.

Choose a chair with arms. Using an armchair when you work at a desk takes the weight of your arms off your shoulders, neck, and back. The best armrest position is close to your body at a height that lets elbows barely touch the armrest as you type at a keyboard, while allowing you to keep your wrist straight and your neck and shoulders relaxed.

LEVEL 3

One-Foot Heel Raise

This is a variation on the heel raises in level 1, but it's more difficult because you stand on one foot instead of two.

1. Start with both feet flat on the floor about hip-width apart, then raise your left foot so it's just off the floor, putting all your weight on the right foot **a**. Hold a chair or counter for balance.

2. Raise yourself on the ball of your right foot so your heel lifts off the floor as high as comfortably possible **b**. Slowly lower back to the floor.

TIP: For an intermediate exercise that bridges two-foot and one-foot heel raises, do two-foot raises holding a light weight.

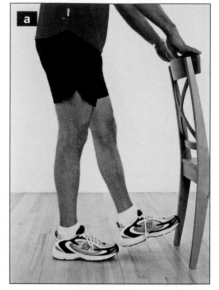

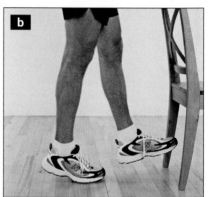

AT THE *Fitness Center*

If you have access to good-quality exercise machines, here's what to use for your ankles and feet:

CALF PRESS MACHINE
If the design of the machine allows, position your feet on the plate so that your heels protrude off the edge, which grants a greater range of motion for this exercise.

MASSAGES

Foot Press

1. Place both hands across the top of your right foot, with your thumbs positioned next to each other on the bottom of the foot **a**.

2. Starting at the heel, use your thumbs to press into the bottom of the foot for one second, then release **b** . Inch your thumbs from your heel toward your toes, pressing and releasing as you go.

3. Do this twice on your right foot and repeat on the other foot.

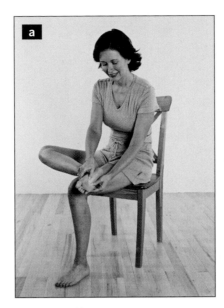

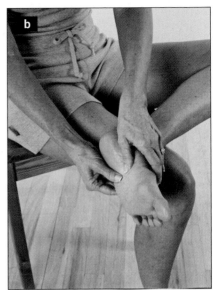

Foot Rocker

1. Start in the same position as the foot press, with hands across the top of your right foot and thumbs on the bottom **a**.

2. Squeeze your foot with your right hand and, while maintaining a firm grasp (not sliding or stroking), twist your hand forward, rotating the foot. (The left hand should remain passive.) **b** Now use the left hand to rotate the foot in the other direction while keeping the right hand passive. Do each motion twice and repeat on the other foot.

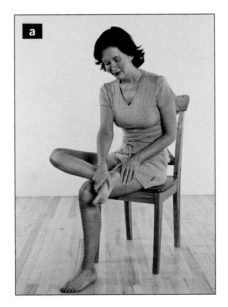

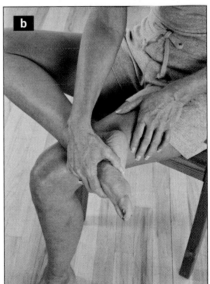

Toe Pull

1. Grasp the tip of your right big toe with the fingers of your left hand and gently pull on the toe while twisting the toe like a knob **a**.

2. Do this twice for each toe on your right foot and repeat on the other foot.

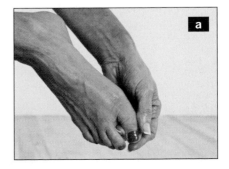

STRETCHES

Arm Hang

This simple exercise is especially useful for improving mobility if you tend to keep elbows bent rather than extending your arms completely—common in people who have lost range of motion due to arthritis.

1. Stand straight with your feet hip-width apart and knees slightly bent.

2. Let your arms hang down by your side and try to straighten them as much as you comfortably can 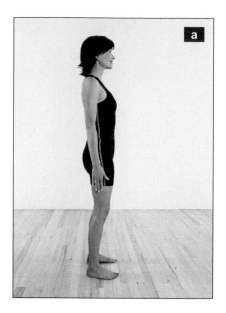. Stop the stretch just prior to locking your elbows. Hold.

TIP: You can also do this stretch while sitting straight on the edge of an armless chair.

Though it's not as common to have arthritis in the elbows as in the hands, knees, and hips, you shouldn't ignore the elbows, which are critically important for all the activities that involve the upper extremities. Increasing strength and flexibility in the elbows translates into improved ability to, say, get out of a chair or to pick up a grandchild. The elbow works with the shoulder and wrist to provide the entire arm with a wide variety of movements, especially if you work to increase its mobility and power.

Forearm Flip

1. Stand straight with your feet hip-width apart and knees slightly bent, arms hanging down by your side. Bend your elbows to 90 degrees with your palms facing upward as if you're holding a tray 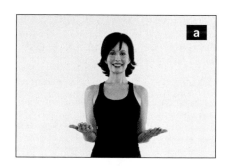. This is your starting position.

2. Smoothly flip your hands over so the palms are facing the floor as much as possible 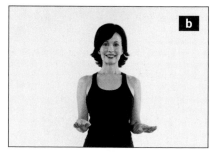. Hold and return to the starting position.

Shoulder Touch

Extending your thumbs in this exercise encourages you to provide more flexion to your elbows, and helps keep your wrists properly aligned.

1. Stand straight with your feet hip-width apart and knees slightly bent, arms hanging down by your side, palms facing your thighs, fingers relaxed, and thumbs pointing to the front **a**.

2. Smoothly bend your elbows, bringing your thumbs toward the same-side shoulders **b**. Hold. Slowly lower your hands back to the starting position.

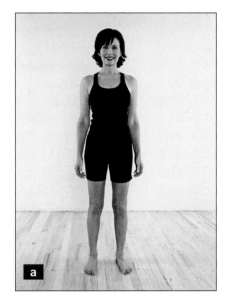

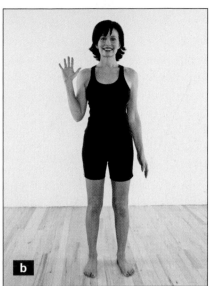

TIP: To maintain proper form, your elbows should remain next to your rib cage through the entire exercise.

STRENGTH EXERCISES

`LEVEL 1`

Seated Biceps Curl

This is a fundamental exercise for the biceps muscles that support the elbow at the front of the upper arm. It's a move that's easily adapted for different degrees of function, and you'll find a variation in all three levels.

1. Sit up straight on the front half of an armless chair, feet flat on the floor, with your arms hanging down by your side **a**.

2. Smoothly bend your elbows, keeping them positioned at your side, raising your hands toward your shoulders while rotating your palms a quarter turn so they face your shoulder at the top of the movement **b**. Smoothly return to the starting position.

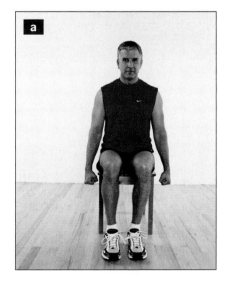

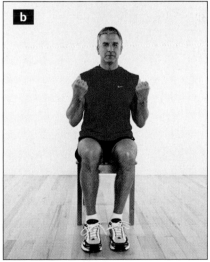

TIP: If you find it difficult or painful to lift your forearms from an extended position, rest your arm next to you on a table or the arm of a chair with your elbow padded by a towel as a starting position. This allows you to avoid the most difficult part of the movement while still working the biceps to increase strength. When you finish one arm, repeat with the other.

Armchair Dip

This is an exercise that encourages you to work muscles exactly the way you use them for everyday activities.

1. Sit in a sturdy armchair, back straight and feet flat on the floor about hip-width apart. Place your hands on the chair's arms about even with the front of your body **a**.

2. Using mostly your arms but assisting with your legs, push yourself out of the chair to a full standing position **b**, letting go of the chair as you stand **c**.

3. Lower yourself back into the chair, putting hands on the arms of

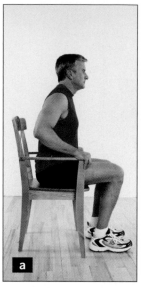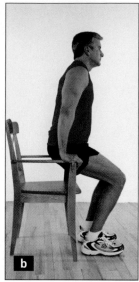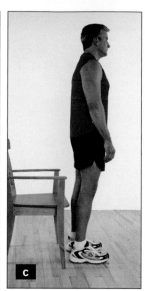

the chair as you slowly come down, using your arm muscles to return to the starting position.

TIP: For a variation maintain your hold on the arms of the chair until you fully extend arms then slowly lower yourself back into the chair.

LEVEL 2

Biceps Curl with Weights

This variation of the biceps curl adds hand weights for resistance. If you have trouble holding them, you can strap weights around your wrists for resistance.

1. Sit up straight on the front half of an armless chair, feet flat on the floor, your arms by your side and a hand weight in each hand **a**.

2. Slowly bend your right elbow, keeping it positioned at your side, raising the weight toward your shoulder while rotating your palm a quarter turn so it faces your shoulder at the top of the movement **b**.

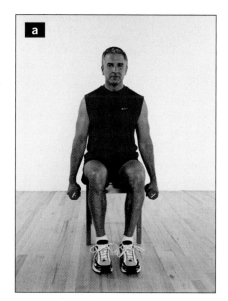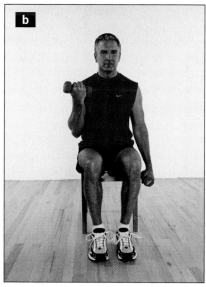

3. Slowly return to the starting position and repeat with the left arm for one repetition.

TIPS:
• Performing this exercise with alternating arms allows each arm to rest momentarily between repetitions.

• As you become stronger, do arms together. As that becomes easier, add weight and use alternating arms.

Hammer Curl

This exercise is similar to the standard biceps curl, but by angling the weight a different way, it also works muscles in the forearm that support the elbow.

1. Sit up straight on the front half of an armless chair, feet flat on the floor, arms hanging down by your sides and a hand weight in each hand, palms facing your thighs **a**.

2. Keeping your elbows close to your sides and your wrists straight, bend your right elbow, raising the weight end-first toward your right shoulder **b**.

3. Hold for one second and slowly return to the starting position. Repeat with the left arm.

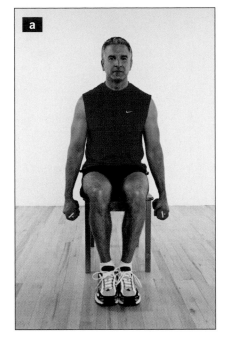

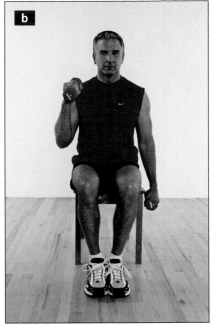

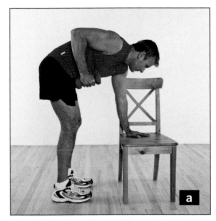

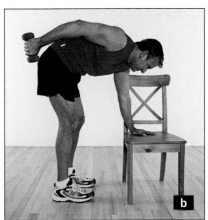

Triceps Kickback

This exercise works the muscles opposite the biceps on the back of your upper arm. If you have trouble holding hand weights, you can strap weights around your wrists for resistance.

1. Stand in front of a chair or bench holding a hand weight in your right hand. Bend forward at the waist, putting your left hand on the chair or bench so you feel stable. Keeping your knees slightly bent, bring your right elbow to your rib cage, so your arm is bent at about 90 degrees and the weight is hanging toward the floor **a**. This is your starting position.

2. Keeping your elbow next to your body, smoothly push the weight behind you, extending your elbow until it is nearly straight (but not locked) **b**.

3. Hold for one second and slowly lower the weight to the starting position. After completing one set, repeat with the left arm.

Elbows >

everyday *secrets*

Leave the pool well. Finish off your water workout by using a fitness trick to get out of the pool. Go to the shallow end and stand with your back against the side of the pool. Reach back to place your palms on the edge of the pool and jump up so that you sit on the edge. Assisted by the buoyancy of your body in the water, this movement works your arms, shoulders, chest, and back.

Park with employees. When shopping at the mall, park where workers are told to put their cars—away from entrances. Better yet, park at the end of the mall farthest from the store to which you're heading and walk to your destination. (Bonus: You'll have no trouble finding a spot.)

Take the long way. Most people try to find the shortest route to where they're going. But if you're hoofing it, short is good but long is better. Think of other ways to decide which way to go. Examples: Which way has more beautiful scenery, less traffic, a coffee shop, attractive stores, or friendly people you might speak with?

continued on page 118

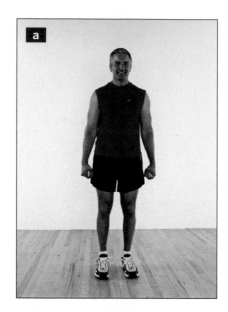

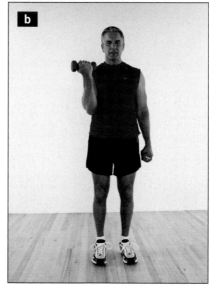

Standing Biceps Curl

By standing in this version of the biceps curl, you work your arm muscles but also call on muscles in the torso and lower body needed to stabilize your balance.

1. Stand straight with your feet hip-width apart and knees slightly bent, holding a hand weight in each hand with arms hanging down by your side, palms facing your thighs **a**.

2. Keeping your right elbow at your side, rotate your hand so your palm faces forward. Bend your elbow to raise the weight toward your shoulder so that your palm faces your shoulder at the top of the lift **b**.

3. Hold for one second and slowly lower the weight to the starting position, turning palms inward as you reach the bottom of the movement.

4. When your right arm is all the way down, repeat with the left arm.

TIP: It's tempting to come down only partway at the end of a biceps curl because the exercise becomes more difficult as your arm straightens. But it's important to bring arms all the way down and complete the wrist rotation at the bottom of every repetition. This momentarily works the biceps from a slightly different direction, making the exercise more effective.

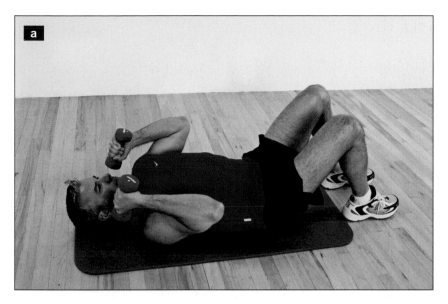

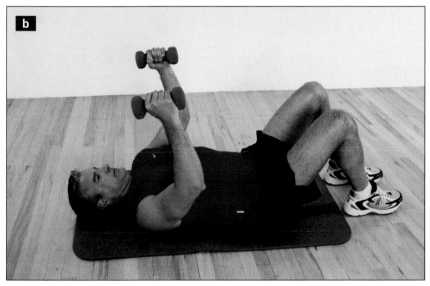

Lying Triceps Extension

1. Lie on the floor or an exercise mat with your knees bent and feet flat on the floor. Hold a hand weight in each hand, placing them vertically on end on the floor next to your ears **a**.

2. Keeping your elbows pointed toward the ceiling, straighten your arms as far as is comfortably possible without locking your elbows, so that knuckles will point toward the ceiling and the bars of the weights are parallel to the floor **b**.

3. Slowly lower the weight back to the floor to complete one repetition.

AT THE *Fitness Center*

If you have access to good-quality exercise machines, here's what to use for your elbows:

SEATED TRICEPS PUSH-DOWN
To effectively work your triceps muscles using this machine, lean forward slightly at the waist to put your body in a better-leveraged position.

ASSISTED DIP
When you press upward to straighten your arms, be sure that your elbows are not locked.

In some ways, the wrist is a forgotten joint when it comes to strength and flexibility. It's easy to assume that if you're exercising the elbows and hands, the wrist is getting a good workout too. In many cases, that's true. But the wrist deserves special attention—and exercises—all its own because it plays an important part in daily functioning. If you splint a painful wrist and lose complete mobility, you'll quickly understand how necessary its movements are. By doing these exercises, you'll make sure your wrist is in tiptop shape.

STRETCHES

Handshake Wrist Bend

1. Stand straight with your feet hip-width apart and knees slightly bent, your arms hanging down by your sides. Bend your elbows 90 degrees so your forearms are parallel to the floor. Point your thumbs up and open your fingers loosely as if you were going to shake someone's hand **a** .

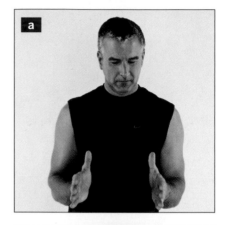

2. Keeping your forearms parallel to the floor, smoothly move your hands to the outside so that your palms are facing as far forward as comfortably possible **b** .

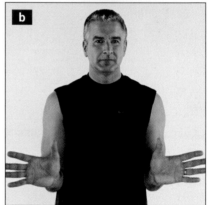

3. Smoothly return to the starting position and move your hands inward as far as comfortably possible so that your palms face your body **c** . Return to the starting position for one repetition. Do six repetitions.

TIP: This is an active stretch, so don't hold your wrists in any given position, but instead keep hands moving.

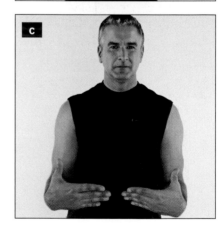

Prayer Stretch

1. Stand straight with your feet hip-width apart and knees slightly bent. Put your palms together in front of your face, elbows down by your side as if praying **a**.

2. Slowly lower your hands in front of your body as your elbows move outward, keeping your fingers pointing up, until you feel a slight stretch in your elbows, forearms, and wrist **b** .

TIP: Don't move your arms lower than necessary to keep forearms parallel to the floor or you'll put more stress on the wrist than is necessary for functional movement.

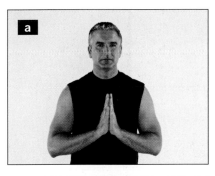

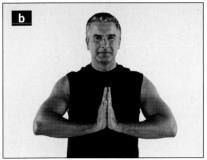

Wrist Circle

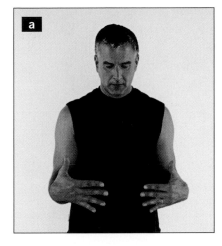

This stretch incorporates all the movements of the wrist in a single continuous motion.

1. Stand straight with your feet hip-width apart and knees slightly bent, with your elbows at your sides and flexed 90 degrees, with thumbs pointing up and fingers open.

2. Move your hands at the wrist to trace large circles with your fingertips, moving in an inward direction **a**. Do 6 repetitions. Repeat in reverse, tracing circles in an outward direction.

Side to Side

1. Stand straight with your feet hip-width apart and knees slightly bent, your elbows at your sides and flexed 90 degrees, palms facing downward.

2. Keeping your fingers parallel to the floor, slowly move your hands outward, then inward, like a gesture you'd make to say, "None of that," for one repetition **a** . Do 5 repetitions.

TIP: If it's more comfortable, you can also do this active stretch with your palms facing upward: Because rotating the open hand comes mostly from the elbow, not the wrist, the muscle action in the wrist is about the same no matter which direction your palms are facing.

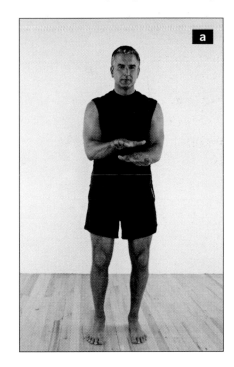

STRENGTH EXERCISES

LEVEL 1

Wrist Curl

This exercise works the wrist along with the entire forearm.

1. Sit in a chair with your forearms resting on your thighs and your hands extended off your knees with your palms facing upward. Relax your hands, allowing your fingers to drop toward the floor. This is your starting position **a**.

2. Slowly bend your wrists to bring your fingers up so they point toward the ceiling as far as is comfortably possible **b**.

3. Slowly lower your fingers back to the starting position for one repetition.

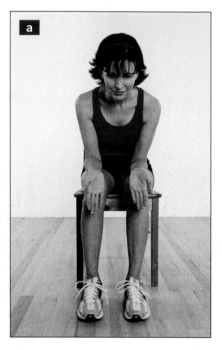

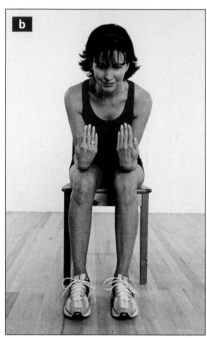

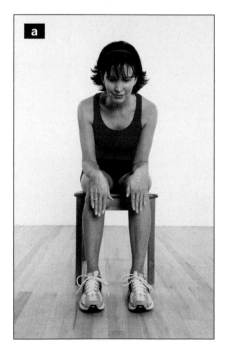

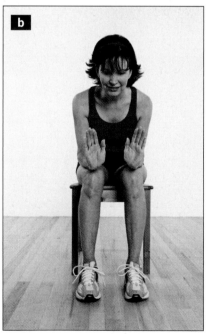

Wrist Extension

Think of this exercise as wrist curls in reverse.

1. Sit in a chair with forearms resting on your thighs and your hands extended over your knee with your palms facing the floor. Relax your wrist so your palms are against the upper part of your shin **a**.

2. Bending at the wrist, lift your hands upward as far as comfortably possible **b**.

3. Slowly lower your hands to the starting position and repeat.

Wrist Rotation

1. Sit in a chair, feet flat on the floor about hip-width apart. Rest your forearms on your thighs and extend your hands over your knees with your palms facing the floor.

2. Make loose fists **a** and, keeping your wrists straight, turn your fists so your palms are up **b**, Then turn them back so your palms are down again for one repetition.

TIP: You could also do this exercise with your hands open, but making a fist keeps the movement cleaner and prepares you for the level-2 version, in which you hold weights.

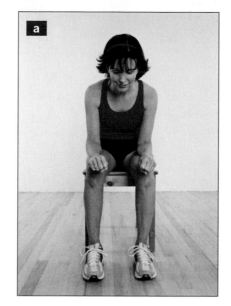 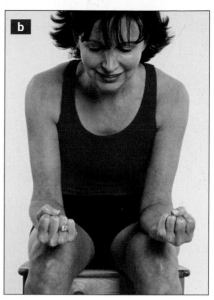

`LEVEL 2`

Weighted Wrist Curl

Performed like the wrist curls in level 1, this exercise is significantly more difficult with hand weights.

1. Sit in a chair holding a weight in each hand, with your forearms resting on your thighs and your hands extended off your knee with your palms facing upward. Relax your hands, allowing the weights to move toward the floor. This is your starting position **a**.

2. Roll your fingers to bring the weights comfortably into your hands. Slowly bend your wrists to bring the weights toward the ceiling as far as is comfortably possible **b**.

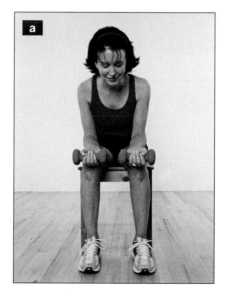 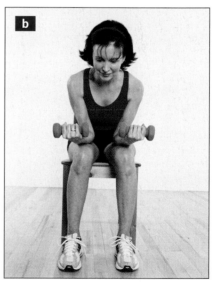

3. Slowly lower the weights back to the starting position for one repetition.

TIP: If you find it difficult to lift both weights together, start by doing alternating curls.

Weighted Wrist Extension

Here, too, the adding of hand weights makes this level-1 motion an exercise with level-2 intensity.

1. Sit in a chair and hold a weight in each hand, with forearms resting on your thighs and your hands extended over your knee with your palms facing the floor. Relax your wrists so the weights are resting against the upper part of your shins **a**.

2. Bending at the wrists, lift the weights upward as far as comfortably possible **b**.

3. Slowly lower your hands to the starting position and repeat.

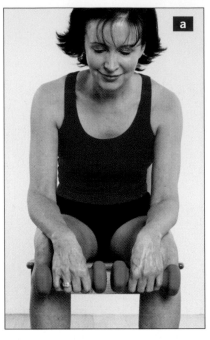

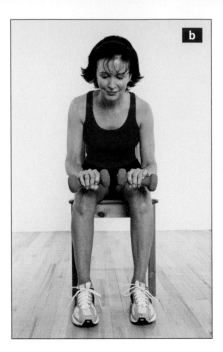

TIP: As with wrist curls, if you find it difficult to lift both weights together, start by alternating hands.

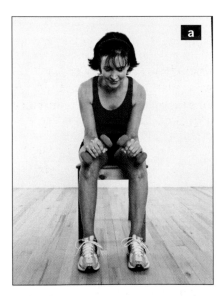

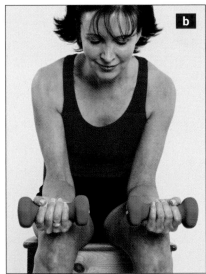

Weighted Wrist Rotation

Performed with hand weights, this exercise is more intense than the version in level 1.

1. Sit in a chair and hold a weight in each hand, forearms resting on your thighs, with palms facing downward and feet flat on the floor about hip-width apart.

2. Keeping your wrists straight, turn your fists **a** so your palms are up **b**, then turn them back so your palms are down again for one repetition.

TIP: If your weights tend to strike or get in each other's way, place your feet slightly farther apart to create more space between your knees.

Standing Wrist Curl

Though it's a curl, this exercise works at a more intense angle than regular curls, isolating muscles of the inner forearm.

1. Stand straight with your feet hip-width apart and your knees slightly bent. Grasp a hand weight in each hand, with your arms by your sides and palms facing behind you **a**.

2. Bend your wrist to curl your hands behind you as far as comfortably possible **b** **c**.

3. Slowly lower your hands to the starting position.

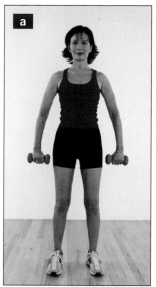
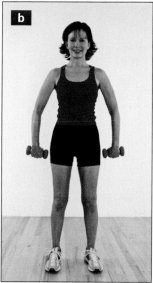
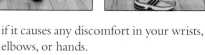

TIP: Before you try this exercise, be sure you can perform the backward-bending wrist movement without resistance to see if it causes any discomfort in your wrists, elbows, or hands.

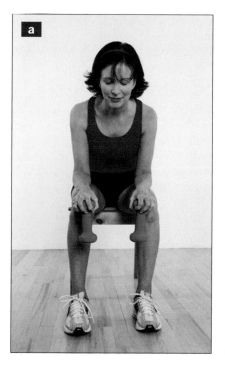

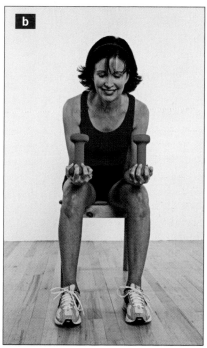

Thor's Hammer

Though the motion is similar to a wrist rotation, the way you hold the weights in this exercise adds considerably more resistance.

1. Sit in a chair and hold a weight in each hand, grasping the weight on one end (not in the middle of the handgrip) with palms facing downward **a**.

2. Keeping your wrists straight, turn the weights so your palms are up **b**. Then rotate hands back so your palms face down.

TIP: Start with a light weight—perhaps weighing 25 percent less than what you used for level-2 wrist curls. Or start with the lightest weight you have and work upward as your condition allows.

STRETCHES

Finger Stretch

This is move is designed to extend your fingers' range of motion.

1. Place one hand on a tabletop or your thigh with your palm facing down.

2. Spread your fingers apart as far as you can, and hold **a** . Repeat with the other hand.

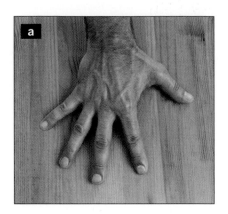

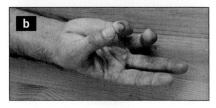

Gentle Fist

1. Place your right hand in a relaxed position, palm up, on a tabletop or your thigh.

2. Roll your fingers in toward your palm so that you make a loose fist. Try to bring your fingers as close together as is comfortable without squeezing **a** . Hold.

3. Release and roll your fingers out to the starting position, and repeat with the other hand.

Thumb Touch

1. Place your hand, palm up, on a table with your fingers open and your hand relaxed.

2. Smoothly move the tip of your thumb into contact with the tip of your index finger, lightly touching, but not pressing them together **a** . Hold for one second. Relax and return to the starting position.

3. In a similar manner, bring your middle finger to your thumb, hold, and return.

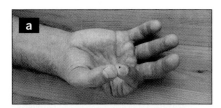

4. Do the same thing for the ring and pinkie fingers, and repeat with the other hand **b** .

Hand joints are among the most common targets of arthritis. Yet because the muscles in the hands are small, you can give yourself a workout appropriate for restoring function with a minimal number of stretches and exercises involving very little resistance. What's more, exercises that you may already have done during your workout often do double duty working the hands. In fact, some of the best exercises for the hands involve movements that are also described in other sections.

STRENGTH EXERCISES

LEVEL 1

Towel Grab

1. Lay a hand towel flat on a table-top. Place your right hand on the edge of the towel palm-down so that your fingers are on the edge of the towel, but the rest of your hand is off it **a**.

2. Slowly pull the towel toward the palm of your hand by bending all four fingers inward **b**. Continue for the entire length of the towel. Repeat with the other hand.

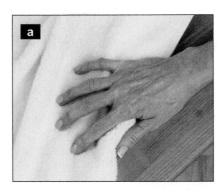 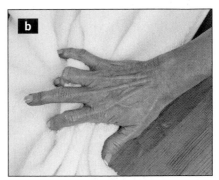

TIP: If arthritis pain or stiffness makes it difficult to pull a hand towel, start with a washcloth. To add resistance, the towel can be dampened with warm water.

Spider Walk

The movement in this exercise is a variation on the towel grab, but the weight of your arm provides more resistance.

1. Place your right hand palm-down on a tabletop **a**.

2. Using your fingers, pull your palms across the table as far as you can comfortably reach **b**. Repeat with the other hand.

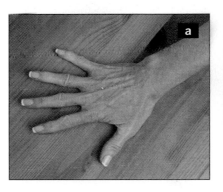 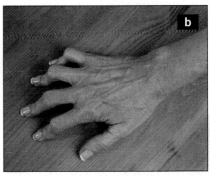

TIP: As you get stronger, add resistance by using fewer fingers to draw your hand across, and alternate the exercise on different fingers to make sure each one gets a workout. Use as many or as few fingers as feels comfortable.

AT THE *Fitness Center*

If you have access to good-quality exercise machines, here's what to use for your hands:

PULL-DOWN MACHINE
The reaching, grasping, and pulling involved with this back exercise (see Back and Spine, page 89) make it an excellent exercise for the hands as well.

Wrist Curl

This exercise is good for the wrist (see also page 112), but uses the muscles of the hands to perform the movement.

1. Sit in a chair with your forearms resting on your thighs and your hands extended off your knees with your palms facing upward. Relax your hands, allowing your fingers to drop toward the floor. This is your starting position.

2. Slowly bend your wrists to bring your fingers up so they point toward the ceiling as far as is comfortably possible **a**.

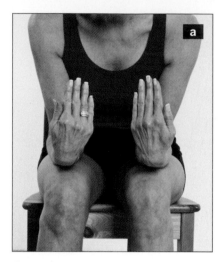

3. Slowly lower your fingers back to the starting position for one repetition.

Wrist Extension

Another exercise that's described in the wrist section (see page 112), this movement also uses the muscles of the hands—but different ones from those used in wrist curls.

1. Sit in a chair with forearms resting on your thighs and your hands extended over your knee with your palms facing the floor. Relax your wrist so your palms are against the upper part of your shin.

2. Bending at the wrist, lift your hands upward as far as comfortably possible **a**.

3. Slowly lower your hands to the starting position and repeat.

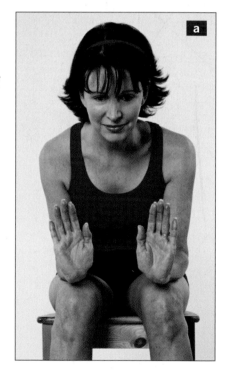

MASSAGES

Palm Stroke

Hold your right palm facing up in your left hand so that your left thumb sits in your right palm **a**. Press the flesh of your palm as you move your thumb in a straight line toward the base of your forefinger **b**. Do the same toward each finger. Do the entire exercise twice and repeat with the other hand.

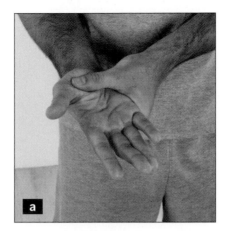

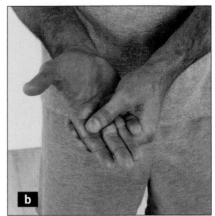

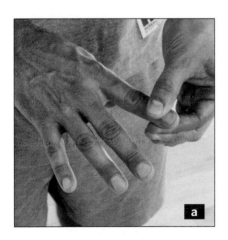

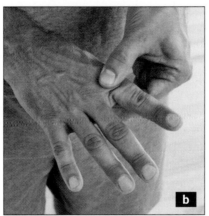

Finger Stroke

Take hold of your right forefinger with all the fingers of your left hand **a**. Starting from the middle knuckle, slide your fingers down the digit toward the base of the finger two times **a**. Then do the same thing from the fingertip to the middle knuckle **b**. Do this for all the fingers, and repeat with the other hand.

Finger Twist

This massage increases both circulation and the motion of the joint.

1. As with finger strokes, take hold of your right forefinger with all the fingers of your left hand, as if you were putting on a ring.

2. Use the fingers of your left hand to twist the right finger like you're turning a knob, while sliding your fingers from the base of the digit to the fingertip **a**.

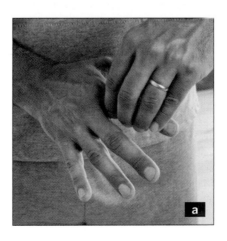

3. Do this twice for each finger and repeat on the other hand.

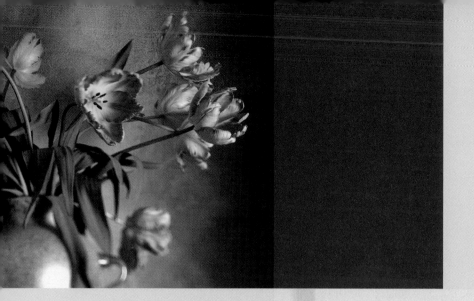

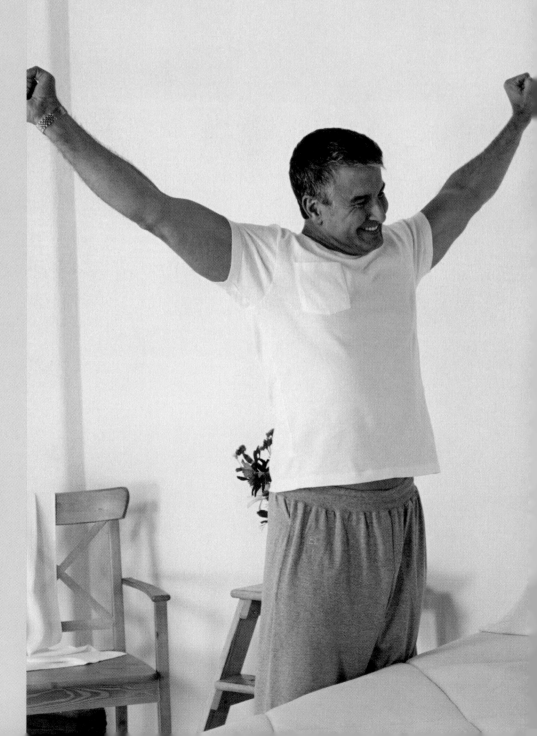

programs for living

Let's say you wanted to put together just five exercises or stretches that are best for you and you alone. Based on the exercises we just detailed in Part III, you would have no less than 9 billion possible combinations! Clearly, you could use some help. ● The programs in this section are specifically designed to address some of the most common objectives of people with arthritis. Plus, we've put together more than 100 tips and secrets for easier living with arthritis.

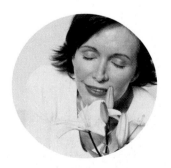

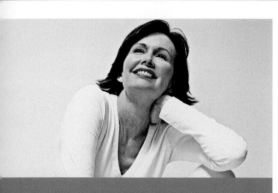

making the
Program Work

Stretching and exercise don't have to be up-and-at-'em activities. This particular routine is gentle, calm, yet comprehensive, so that by the time your feet hit the floor, you've done a body-wide sequence of movements that will make it easier to carry on with your day. The exercises are designed to hit areas that are crucial for the mobility and dexterity you'll need to get through your morning routine. If you worry that your function level is lower in the morning than later in the day, rest assured that each of these stretches and exercises is appropriate for all but the most severe amounts of stiffness.

For many people with arthritis, mornings are the toughest time. Even after a restful night of sleep, the morning hours bring stiffness and pain.

For mornings like these, here is a gentle, eight-step exercise sequence to be done right in bed, right after you awaken.

Remember: No matter how much you wish to resist, moving your body is the best thing you can do. As you use joints and muscles, they loosen up and make the rest of your day easier. This routine, which mixes gentle stretches with simple strengthening moves, gives you an easy start that gradually makes further movement more manageable.

Instructions

For the stretches, hold your position for 15 seconds before releasing. For the strength exercises, do one set of 6 repetitions. Rest 30 seconds between each movement. Remain lying for the first three, then raise yourself to a sitting position for the rest. Move slowly and smoothly in a relaxed and gentle manner without a lot of abrupt motions. This ensures you'll gradually increase blood supply to stiff joints and supporting structures, warming them up and making them supple.

> The Morning Routine

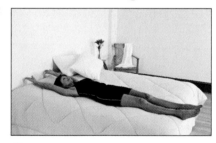

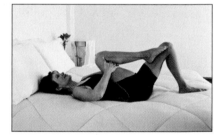

1. Lying Total Body Stretch

Without getting up, stretch your arms and legs to get blood flowing throughout your body. **Page 77**

2. Low Back Knees to Chest

Push the covers off if you haven't already, and slowly bring your knees to your chest. Return and repeat. This will help your back and hips. **Page 82**

Getting Out of Bed

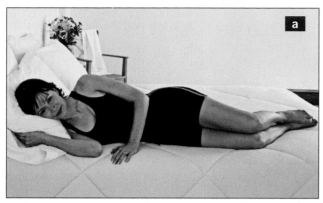

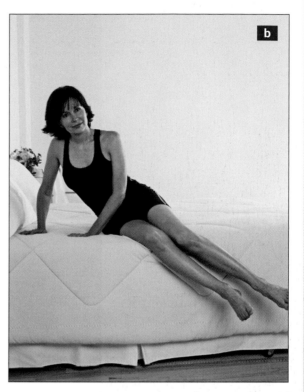

If back pain or other aches make getting out of bed in the morning a challenge, follow this technique.

1. First, roll onto your side, facing the edge of the bed **a**.

2. Next swing your legs out over the edge. Then push your body up with your arms until you're in a sitting position on the edge of the bed **b**.

3. Finally, stand up solidly on both feet.

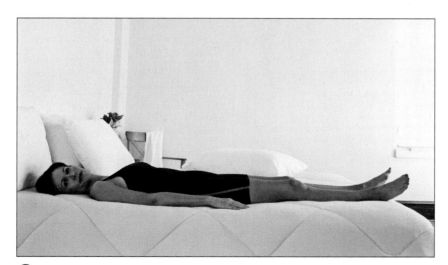

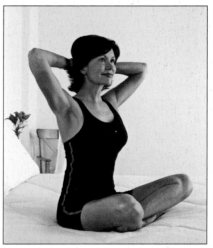

3. Neck Turn

While still lying down, gently stretch your neck muscles right and then left to ease tension in your head, neck, and shoulders. **Page 94**

4. Seated Chest Stretch

Lengthen your chest muscles with this simple, pleasing stretch. **Page 90**

Program continues >

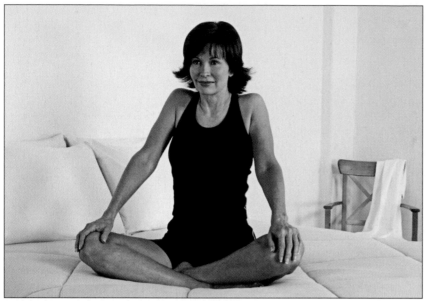

5. Shoulder Roll

Another soothing motion for your head, neck, and shoulders. **Page 68**

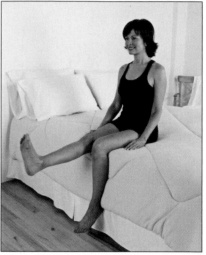

6. Seated Knee Extension

Slowly sit up for this stretch.
Page 52

everyday *secrets*

THE NIGHTTIME ROUTINE

Do a pre-sleep stretch. Stretching isn't just for the morning: Studies of patients with rheumatoid arthritis show that 15 minutes of stretching before you go to bed can significantly ease stiffness the next morning.

Prepare for nighttime nature calls. Make sure you clear a pathway to the bathroom that you can easily navigate in the dark before you go to bed. Keep doors fully opened or fully closed so you don't run into the edge. And even if you don't use a cane, walker, or other assistance device during the day, consider keeping one by your bed at night to help ensure you keep your balance and detect obstacles when you're stiff and in the dark.

Take analgesics early. If you wake up early (perhaps to use the bathroom), take your pain-relieving medicine and go back to bed. This gives the drug time to kick in so that it's up to full strength when you actually get up to start your day.

Get hot in bed. If you have an electric blanket, turn up the heat just after waking to warm joints and help relieve morning stiffness.

Handle bed height. Mattresses today are much higher than in the past, which is a problem if it forces you to hop down from a height. Ways to manage meaty mattresses:

• Place a folding step stool with a handle next to the bed so you can climb down off the bed without putting extra strain on your joints.

• Get a platform bed that requires just a mattress, eliminating the extra height of a box spring.

Don comfy clothes. Putting on an extra layer of clothing as soon as you get out of bed may help you warm your joints faster. A sweatshirt and sweatpants would be a good bet, but if you find it difficult to pull them on, try putting on a fleece vest or a sweatshirt that zips. Another option: a bathrobe made of thick terry cloth, chamois, or wool.

Choose practical slippers. Slippers without a back are easier to get in and out of than heel-covering styles. But backless slippers are more difficult to keep on when going up and down stairs.

THE MORNING ROUTINE

Get a grip. The trick to taking the discomfort out of manipulating thin toothbrush handles is to beef up the grip. Ways to make your oral hygiene more effective:

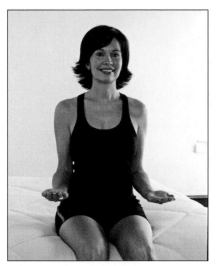

7. Forearm Flip

Now give your elbows some relief and exercise with this gentle movement. **Page 104**

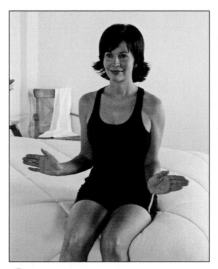

8. Wrist Circle

End the sequence with these gentle moves to ready your hands and wrists for washing, brushing your teeth, and preparing breakfast. **Page 111**

Enter the Shower Safely

The best bet for getting in and out: Use a shower stall instead of a bathtub, which allows you to simply walk into the shower without lifting your legs over the edge of a tub. But when dealing with a tub, start by getting in at the end farthest from the faucet or shower head, which is likely to be a bit drier, warmer, and less slippery. Stand with your hip to the side of the tub, bend the knee closest to the tub, keeping your upper leg straight so that you raise your foot behind you, then swing your foot into the tub and bring your other foot over the same way.

• Wrap your toothbrush in slip-on grips, spongy tape, or other materials that hardware or medical specialty stores may offer to make handles thicker. Ad hoc alternative: Wrap handles in foam hair curlers or a sponge.

• Get an electric toothbrush, which will have a thick plastic handle (where batteries are typically stored) and doesn't require vigorous hand motion to give your teeth a thorough cleaning.

Tackle toothpaste. When painful, stiff, or weak hands make squeezing the toothpaste tube difficult, let your fingers off the hook. Put the tube down on the counter and lean on it gently with the heel of your palm or even your elbow to squeeze out a small amount of paste and apply it to your brush.

Focus on fixtures. Ease discomfort from turning on the water by installing handles that extend and can be grabbed with your entire hand rather than compact handles that must be twisted with your fingers.

Manage medicine lids. If there are no children or grandchildren in the house, ask your pharmacist to fill your prescription using non-childproof lids, which screw or lift off like they did in the old days. If kid safety is an issue, ask a family member or friend to help sort your medications into a weekly dispenser with a handy flip-top compartment containing pills for each day of the week.

Take a shower. The heat and rush of water soothe joints and muscles, and help your whole body relax, so it's important that the bath or shower itself doesn't become more of an obstacle or source of discomfort than necessary. Basic arthritis-friendly fixtures for easier, safer bathing include:

• Nonskid bath mats to provide sure footing both in the tub or shower stall and the neighboring tile floor. As an added precaution, you can also wear the grip-soled water shoes you may already have for a pool exercise class.

• Bars you can grab to keep your balance and push or pull on while getting in or out.

• A shower seat where you can sit if you get fatigued. If there's not one built into the shower, consider using a folding beach chair or campstool.

• A handheld shower nozzle that can direct water at any angle. If you have a nozzle installed, have the plumber put it at waist height so it's easy to lift on and off. ■

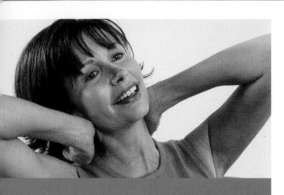

It's tempting just to stretch muscles supporting joints that hurt. But taking that approach would be a mistake. Good flexibility is something *every* joint needs for greater mobility and better posture. Plus, stretched muscles ease tension and take pressure off joints throughout your body.

This program is designed to improve body-wide flexibility with a mix of stretches that hit all your major joints and muscles. Don't be daunted by the 14-stretch sequence. Each exercise takes 15 to 60 seconds, so you can easily do this entire routine in just 5 to 10 minutes, plus a warmup.

Instructions

Begin with 5 to 10 minutes of easy walking or some other light activity to warm up your muscles, tendons, and ligaments. This makes stretches both safer and more effective. Perform the stretches as described in Part III, holding each stretch according to the guidelines for your function level. Flow from one stretch to the other without much pause.

The Stretch Sequence

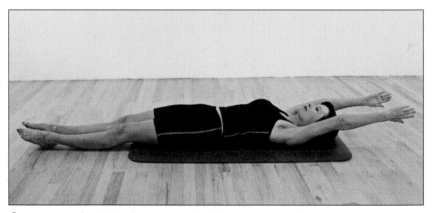

1. Lying Total Body Stretch

This stretch feels great and expands your whole body. It is particularly good for your shoulders and abdomen. **Page 77**

making the
Program Work

It's not harmful to do these stretches in a different order, or to make substitutions for any that feel uncomfortable. But going through the program as outlined has a number of benefits. The idea is to start with a gentle movement that stretches the entire body all at once, then proceed from larger muscles or groups of muscles to smaller or more isolated ones.

The program also keeps exercises moving from one area of the body to another so that stretching activity is evenly distributed as you go. Stretches for muscles that tend to be less pliable in most people (such as the hamstrings in the seated V) are placed so that easier stretches can first prep the area with some preliminary limbering. The workout finishes with a posture exercise that will keep you standing tall even as you move on with your day.

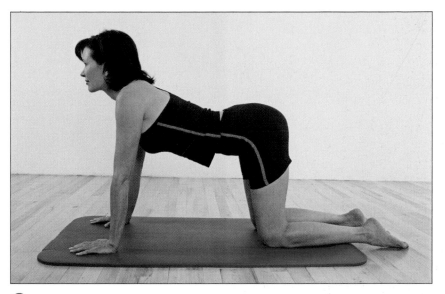

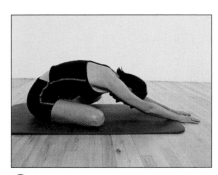

2. Cross-Legged Seated Stretch

Sit up now for a soothing stretch that benefits your lower back. **Page 84**

3. Cat Stretch

Gently pull yourself forward onto your hands and knees for another great stretch for your back. **Page 84**

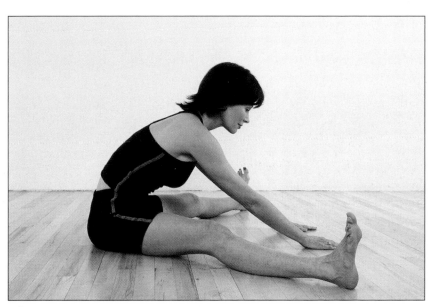

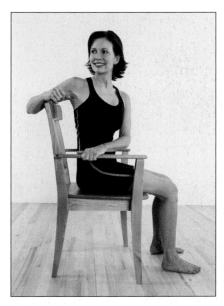

4. Seated V

Now plop back down on your butt, stretch your legs out in front of you, and reach! This stretch helps your knees, hips, and back. **Page 53**

5. Seated Torso Twist

In a chair, stretch your abdomen muscles for better posture and back support. **Page 76**

Program continues >

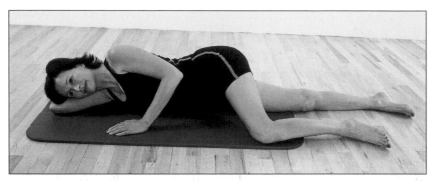

6. Lying Pelvis Rotation

Relax onto the ground and give your hips some relief with this gentle torso stretch. **Page 55**

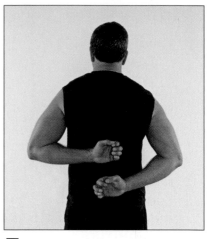

7. Knuckle Rub

Now to your upper body: Work out the tension in your shoulder and neck muscles. You should feel this one deeply. **Page 69**

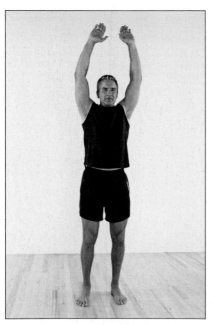

8. "Good Morning" Exercise

Say hello to the world with this soothing shoulder stretch. **Page 70**

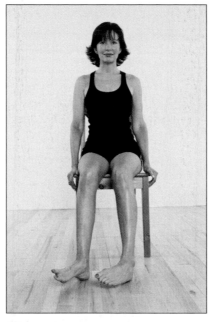

9. Ankle Circle

Gentle foot rotations will help your ankles cope with the day's travels. **Page 98**

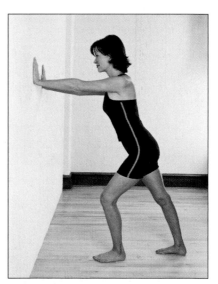

10. Runner's Calf Stretch

This popular stretch does wonders for that important muscle that connects your knee to your ankle. **Page 99**

everyday *secrets*

STRETCHING

Breathe deep. Make your stretching even more relaxing and pain relieving by working in elements of meditation. Specifically, try these simple breathing techniques:

• Breathe through your nose both when inhaling and exhaling.

• Focus on the hiss of air flowing in and out of your nostrils; the calming tone soothes your thoughts.

• Take at least three seconds to fill your lungs and another three to let air out.

Unclench your stretch. Stretching should relax all of you. Don't let your jaw, shoulders, hands, and feet tense up during your routine. Tense body parts make stretching other areas less effective.

Get an extra stretch. The rule of thumb is to stretch until you feel a gentle tug in the muscle. But if that feeling subsides as you hold, are you stretching far enough? The answer is yes—for the 15 seconds or so it takes your muscles to relax with the stretch. That might be enough for you. But if you feel limber enough to push a little farther, stretch another fraction of an inch after you've held for 15 seconds,

then hold for another 15 seconds. This extra push, sometimes called the developmental stretch, helps promote flexibility faster than the first stretch alone.

Keep it up. Even if you don't do other aerobic or strength exercises, it's worth stretching every day: Lengthened muscles only keep their newfound flexibility for a day or less. Consistently working them every day, however, makes them progressively more pliable—as long as you keep stretching. Plus, stretching is good for stress relief and your attitude—every day. ∎

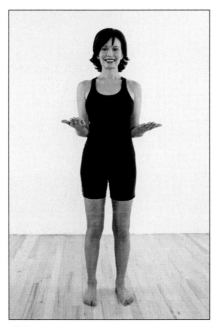

11. Forearm Flip

Almost done. Now do this gentle but important stretch for your elbow. **Page 104**

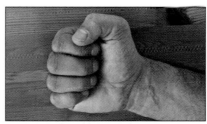

12. Gentle Fist

Bring blood into those fingers and stretch those hand muscles with this simple, reflexive movement. **Page 116**

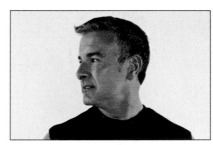

13. Neck Turn

Amazing how much tension finds its way into your neck muscles. These turns offer quick relief. **Page 94**

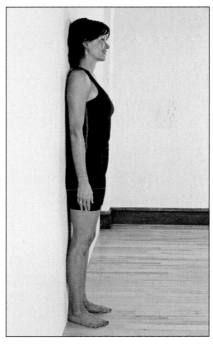

14. Standing Posture Exercise

Conclude this refreshing sequence with a slow, energizing stretch for the spine. **Page 82**

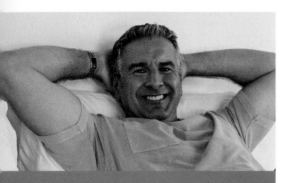

Imagine a strength-training workout that only exercised your arms. You'd find it easy to lift groceries out of the trunk—

but if your legs were weak, you'd have trouble hauling the load up the stairs. Exercise needs to be balanced to make sure your whole body—not just one part—becomes stronger and more mobile. While selected exercises can bolster specific joints, it's important to establish a foundation of strength in all your major muscles that targeted workouts can build upon.

Instructions

You will find three different routines on the following pages: beginning, intermediate, and advanced. On page 134, we give details on how to increase the challenge within each routine as you get stronger. And when you feel like you've mastered one routine, proceed to the next! For each exercise listed, do the following number of repetitions the first time you attempt the program.

> **Beginning:** Do one set of six repetitions.

> **Intermediate:** Do one set of six to eight repetitions.

> **Advanced:** Do one set of eight repetitions.

> BEGINNING Strength Program

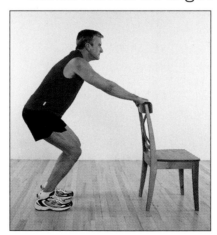

1. Partial Squat

Start your workout with this simple exercise for the hips and thighs. **Level 1, page 57**

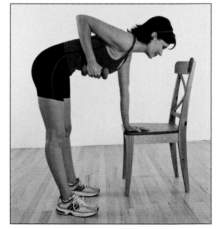

2. Bent Single Arm Row

It would seem like this is an arm exercise, but it is your back muscles doing the work. **Level 2, page 88**

making the Program Work

The basic pattern of a strength workout is to alternate exercises between upper and lower extremities, the front and back of the body, or pushing and pulling motions—all of which allow freshly worked muscles to rest while you hit another area. As you progress through the workouts, you generally go from larger muscles or groups of muscles to smaller ones, with abdominal exercises in the middle to break things up. While each workout targets all the major muscles, a greater number of exercises are devoted to the lower body, which has more muscles that are critical for overall mobility.

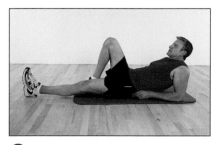

3. Heel Slide

Back to your lower body with this exercise for knees and hips. **Level 1, page 58**

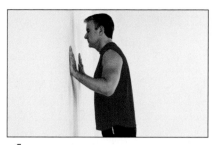

4. Wall Push-Up

This stand-up alternative to the classic exercise is a great way to gently strengthen your chest. **Level 1, page 91**

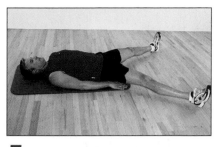

5. Lying Hip Abduction

Get out your mat and on your back to give some exercise to your hips. **Level 1, page 57**

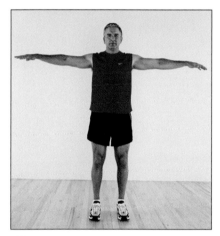

6. Around the World

Get your shoulders moving gently and steadily for suppleness and strength. **Level 2, page 74**

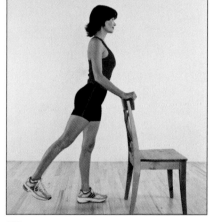

7. Standing Hip Extension

Your hip muscles just got a rest; let's get them moving again. **Level 1, page 60**

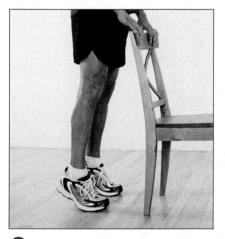

8. Heel Raise

Now exercise your ankles and feet. **Level 1, page 100**

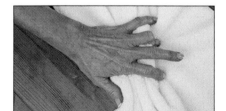

9. Towel Grab

Can't forget the hand and finger muscles. Do 2 repetitions of this exercise with a 30-second break in between reps. **Level 1, page 117**

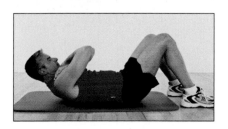

10. Basic Abdominal Curl

Down one more time for this classic exercise. If too tough, do the level 1 modified curl instead. **Level 2, page 78**

> INTERMEDIATE Strength Program

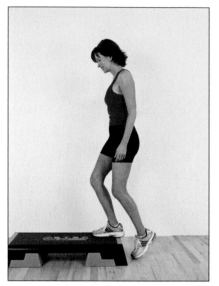

1. Stair Step-Up

Six to eight of these on each side will give your knees and hips a good workout. **Level 2, page 61**

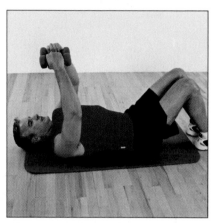

2. Weighted Chest Fly

As your legs rest, here is a great exercise for your chest muscles. **Level 2, page 92**

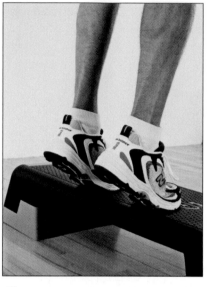

3. Stair Heel Raise

Back to your step for this subtle but useful exercise for ankles and feet. **Level 2, page 100**

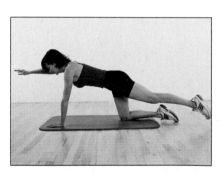

4. Bird Dog

Down on the floor now for this natural strengthener for hips and back. **Level 2, page 62**

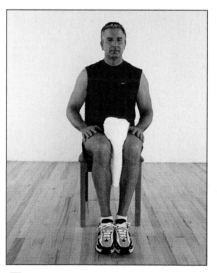

5. Towel Squeeze

It seems so simple, but this exercise really does strengthen your hips. **Level 1, page 58**

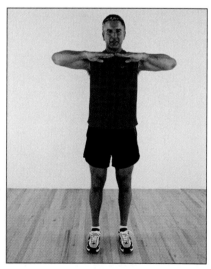

6. Upright Row

Another natural move that, when done in repetition, builds up muscles. **Level 2, page 73**

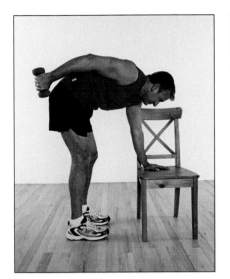

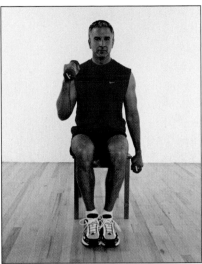

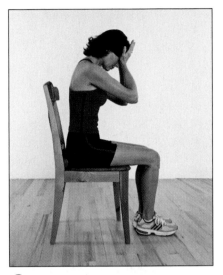

7. Triceps Kickback

Triceps don't get much exercise, so be ready for the challenge! **Level 2, page 107**

8. Hammer Curl

The classic exercise for bigger biceps is also wonderful for your elbow. **Level 2, page 107**

9. "Yes" Exercise

This agreeable exercise is great for your neck (and your attitude). **All levels, page 95**

Program continues >

everyday *secrets*

STRENGTHENING

Book yourself. Don't have time for all this exercise? Sometimes it's a matter of perception—other people's. If coworkers, friends, or even family can't understand why you take time for exercise but not for what they think is important, keep your priorities to yourself—but schedule your exercise in your date book. That way, when sticking to your guns on workouts, you can merely say you're keeping a prior appointment.

Keep it interesting. Some people have a high tolerance for routine—and may even elevate it to ritual. But if your attention span is closer to monkey than monk, try to introduce variety into your workout on a regular basis. One way to do it: Change two things about your routine every week. It could be as simple as adding repetitions, resistance, or sets—or substituting one exercise for another. Change isn't just an antidote to boredom, it allows you to continually challenge muscles in new ways, which makes you stronger faster.

Try slow motion. Want to try a difficult challenge that's easy on joints? Lift a light weight only one time—but do it very slowly. Pick out a weight about half what you'd normally lift 10 times. Take 15 to 20 seconds to lift the weight, hold for another 15 to 20 seconds, then take another 15 to 20 seconds to bring it back down. The constant stress through the entire range of motion will work muscles in an entirely new way.

Judge gym transit time. Made the decision to join a health club? When choosing, follow the golden rule of gym location: Keep it within a 15-minute drive. Any farther and your chances of actually getting there for a workout drop considerably.

Spread the effort. If doing an entire full-body workout all at once is too fatiguing or demanding on your time, try doing only one part of the workout each day. If your workout has 12 exercises,

continued on pg 136

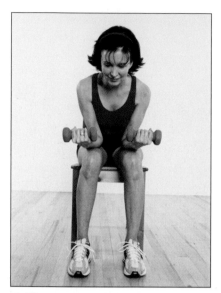

10. Weighted Wrist Curl

This small move is harder than you'd expect, since we rarely test our forearm muscles. **Level 2, page 113**

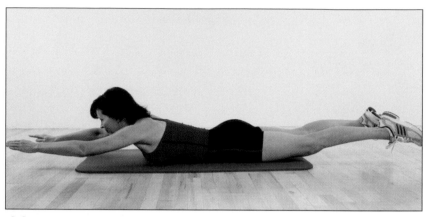

11. Superman

Another feel-good exercise, this time for a healthier and stronger back.
Level 2, page 87

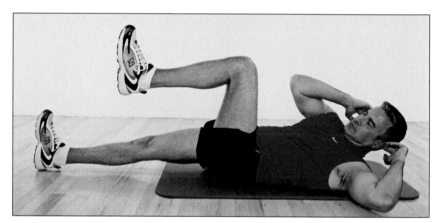

12. Basic Bicycle

End your workout with this youthful move for your abdomen. **Level 2, page 79**

As You Get Stronger

Here is how to progress as you get better with your exercises:

> When you feel comfortable doing the number of starting repetitions, add no more than 1 repetition each time you work out. For example, if you start with 1 set of 6 reps, you could do 1 set of 7 reps next time—or stay at 6 reps if that's still challenging.

> Advance by adding 1 repetition at a time until you can do 12 reps of upper-body exercises, and 15 of lower-body exercises. Continue with that number for two or three consecutive workouts.

> In your next workout, do 1 set of 8 repetitions, rest one to two minutes, then do a second set of 8 repetitions for a total of 16 repetitions. Alternative:

increase the amount of weight (in non-body-weight exercises where you can adjust resistance) by the smallest amount possible (probably 1 pound) and go back to the number of starting reps.

> Continue progressing, changing either the number of sets or amount of resistance (but not both at once) as you go get stronger.

> ADVANCED Strength Program

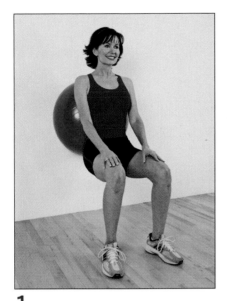

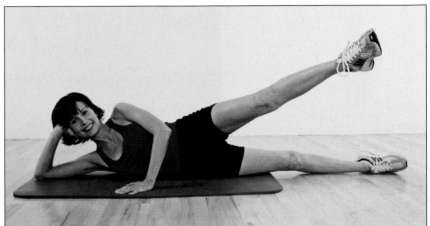

1. Ball Squat

If you don't have an exercise ball, do regular squats. **Level 3, page 63**

2. Side Thrust Kick

This challenges a different set of leg muscles, but aids those same knees and hips. **Level 3, page 63**

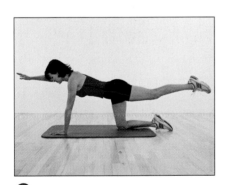

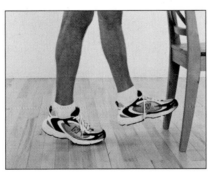

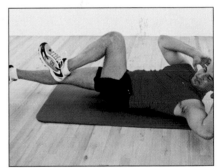

3. Advanced Bird Dog

S-t-r-e-e-e-t-c-h and strengthen your hips and back with this fun exercise. **Level 3, page 65**

4. One-Foot Heel Raise

Strengthen your ankles and feet and improve your balance with this one. **Level 3, page 102**

5. Advanced Bicycle

This abdominal muscle builder will help you transition from lower- to upper-body exercises. **Level 3, page 81**

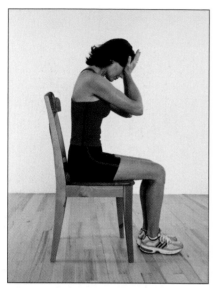 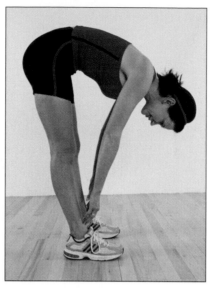 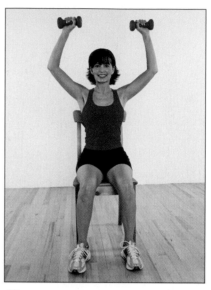

6. "Yes" Exercise

Not as strenuous, but still an important strengthener for the often-neglected neck muscles. **All levels, page 95**

7. Dead Lift

An Olympic-level test! But for you, slow, easy, and smooth for a better back. **Level 3, page 88**

8. Overhead Dumbbell Press

Another classic exercise for strength builders, this for your shoulders. **Level 3, page 75**

continued from page 133

for example, do the first three on Monday, the next three on Tuesday, and the rest on Wednesday. On Thursday, start the routine again. That way, you're still doing each exercise three times during a one-week period without exhausting yourself with your routine.

Hold on to your gains. While giving your muscles a chance to rest is important to making them stronger, there's inevitably a point of diminishing returns when it comes to slacking off. How much rest is too much? A good rule of thumb is to expect about a 10 percent loss of your strength gains after about 10 days. The more training you've done, the slower your strength will decline. The bottom line: To maintain your gains, you need to keep exercising regularly.

Count backward. Problem: Strength exercises are no fun when the last repetitions are tough to do. Interpretation: If you're challenging your muscles enough to want to quit, you're probably doing them at just the right intensity. Mental trick: Your final repetitions will seem easier if you count backward from your target instead of forward from zero because you'll be thinking about how few you have left, rather than how many you've already done.

Get off the floor safely. For exercises and stretches that require you to get on all fours, it's easier to get back up again if you walk your hands back until you're in a kneeling position, place one foot on the floor in front of you with your knee bent at about 90 degrees, then use your leg as a support for your hands as you stand or ease yourself into a chair. ■

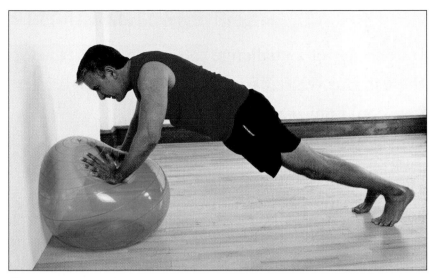

9. Ball Push-Up

A great exercise for your chest. Feel proud if you can do eight good ones. **Level 3, page 93**

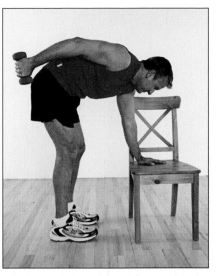

10. Triceps Kickback

It looks so simple and natural, but this arm exercise can be challenging. **Level 2, page 107**

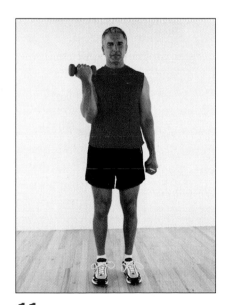

11. Standing Biceps Curl

Don't think about your biceps; think about a better-supported elbow joint. **Level 3, page 108**

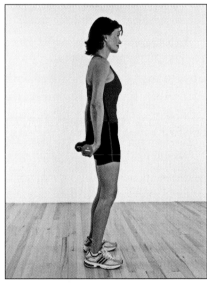

12. Standing Wrist Curl

End this strengthening routine with this simple move for healthier wrists and hands. **Level 3, page 115**

At the Fitness Center

Want a total strengthening program using the machines at the health center? These are the 12 exercises we recommend. Start with two sets of six repetitions of each, and work up from there. Do in the order listed:

1. Leg Press
2. Knee Flexion
3. Machine Abduction/Adduction
4. Pull-Down
5. Chest Press
6. One-Foot Heel Raise
7. Machine Overhead Press
8. Standing Biceps Curl
9. Seated Triceps Pushdown
10. Weighted Wrist Extension
11. Ball Curl
12. Weighted Wrist Rotation

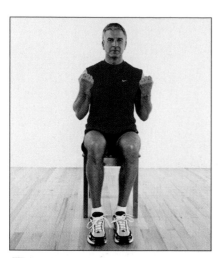

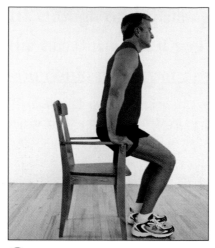

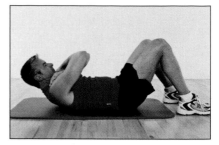

7. Seated Biceps Curl

The classic weightlifting move! But strong biceps aren't just for show—they make carrying things easy and support your elbow. **Level 1, page 105**

8. Armchair Dip

Behind the biceps muscle is the triceps. This exercise strengthens that muscle and also aids your elbows. **Level 1, page 106**

9. Basic or Advanced Abdominal Curl

Remember: Abs exercises don't reduce abdominal fat. But strong abs support your back and make lifting easier. **Level 2 or 3 depending on variation, page 78 or 80**

everyday *secrets*

BURNING CALORIES

Get on the vacuum program. Make vacuuming a total body exercise by stepping forward in a slightly longer-than-usual stride as you move the carpet machine forward while keeping your back straight, then stepping back as you draw the unit toward you again. At the same time you work the muscles of your legs with this lunge-like motion, roll the vacuum cleaner forward with your arms, which uses your shoulder, chest, arm, and upper back for a near-complete workout that contains elements of both strength and aerobic conditioning.

Make every movement count. Fidgeting burns hundreds of calories a day, according to studies at the Mayo Clinic in Rochester, Minnesota, and even chewing gum eats up 11 calories an hour. So don't lose sight of the fact that any form of physical activity—no matter how small—helps your body burn calories. More ways to get movement into your everyday life:

• Always stand up and walk around when on the telephone.

• Always stand up and walk around during television commercials.

• Chop your vegetables by hand, rather than using a food processor.

• While in the car, roll your shoulders and stretch your arms at red lights.

> **INTERMEDIATE** Strength Program   Starting point: 1 set of 6 to 8 repetitions.

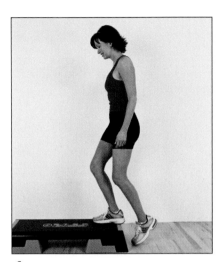

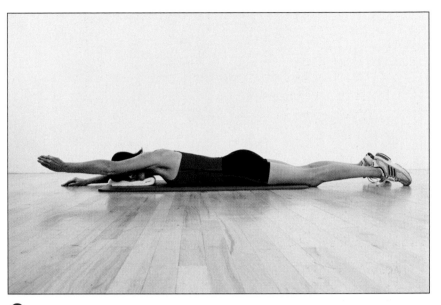

1. Stair Step-Up

By strengthening your thigh muscles with stair step-ups, you take strain off your knees and hips. This is a particularly efficient exercise. **Level 2 or 3, page 61**

2. Lying Alternating Arm Raise

Down on the ground for this simple, wonderful exercise for your back (yes, it is the back muscle pulling your arm up!). **Level 1, page 86**

Program continues >

• Whenever you have music on, tap your toes or bounce your knee to the rhythm.

• Insist on bagging your own groceries at the food store.

Get two workouts in one. You can burn a substantial amount of extra calories during a strength workout if you move quickly from one exercise to the next. By keeping in motion rather than resting between exercises, you are combining strengthening with aerobic exercise, greatly boosting your energy burn. Key trick: Alternate between upper- and lower-body moves, so you give just-exercised muscles time to rest.

Track your metabolism. Even if you boost your metabolism, how would you know? It's largely been a matter of guesswork or cumulative results on the bathroom scale. Now, however, health providers and fitness centers can help clients track their resting metabolic rate (RMR)—the basic measure of metabolism—using a new device called the BodyGem. When you breathe into the handheld inhaler-like unit for a few minutes, your current RMR pops up on a digital readout, giving you a calorie goal for both diet and exercise—and a tangible way to check on your progress. To find healthcare professionals or gyms using the BodyGem, check a locator feature on the manufacturer's website, www.healthetech.com. ■

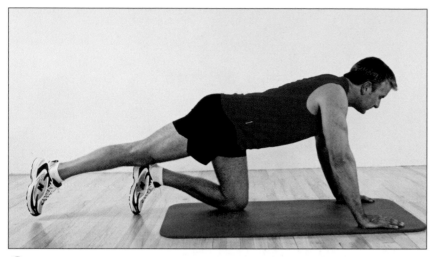

3. Lower-Body Extension

Another gentle yet effective strengthening move for your hips and back.
Level 1, page 59

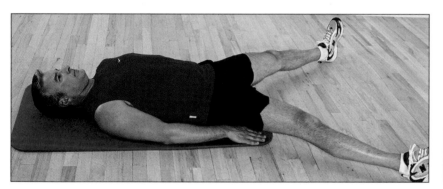

4. Lying Hip Abduction

Give yourself space and move slowly to do this terrific hip exercise
properly. **Level 1, page 57**

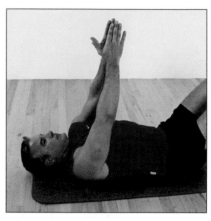

5. Chest Fly

You might be surprised how this
seemingly natural move gives your
chest muscles a good workout.
Level 1, page 92

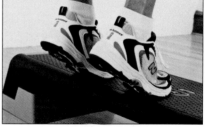

6. Stair Heel Raise

By doing this on a stair, you
lengthen the upward and downward movement, giving an even
better workout for your calves, ankles and feet. **Level 2, page 100**

Aerobic Program

Do your aerobic activity 4 to 6
days a week, progressing as
your comfort level allows, following these guidelines:

> If you're new to cardiovascu-
lar exercise, begin by walking
2 minutes at a slow, leisurely
pace followed by 1 to 2 minutes of brisk walking.

> Once you're comfortable ex-
ercising for a total of 5 minutes, gradually boost the brisk
walking period by 30 to 60
seconds per week.

> Build up gradually to a rou-
tine in which you walk at a
leisurely pace for 2 to 5 minutes, then walk briskly the rest
of the time. Build your total
walking time to between 20
and 40 minutes.

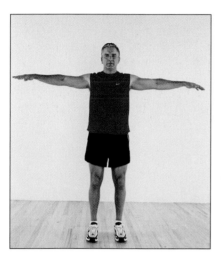

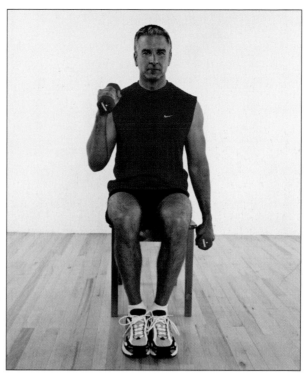

7. Around the World

Feel like a child again with these large but precise arm movements that aid your shoulders. **Level 2, page 74**

8. Hammer Curl

A slight twist on the standard biceps curl that offers a greater challenge to your largest arm muscle. **Level 2, page 107**

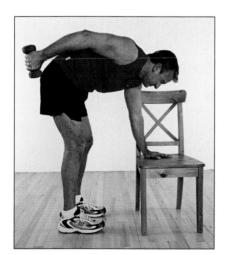

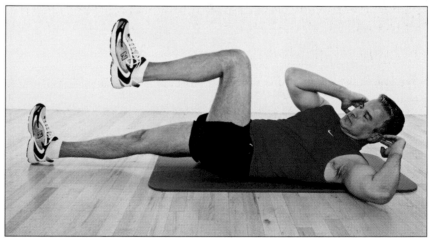

9. Triceps Kickback

Triceps are often much weaker than your biceps, so do this gently and carefully and don't push too hard at first. **Level 2, page 107**

10. Basic or Advanced Bicycle

Great for your abs, but also a wonderful calorie burner. **Level 2 or 3 depending on variation, page 79 or 81**

> ADVANCED Strength Program

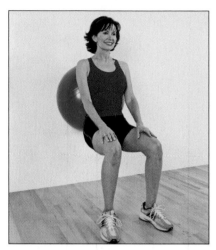 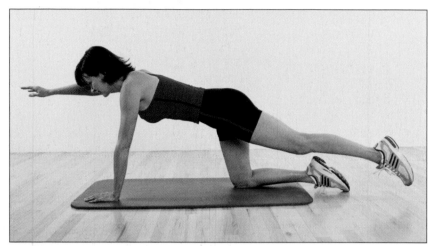

1. Ball Squat

A challenging first exercise that tests your thigh muscles and supports your knees and hips. **Level 3, page 63**

2. Bird Dog

Now onto your hands and knees for this leg-extending exercise that supports your hips and back. **Level 2, page 62**

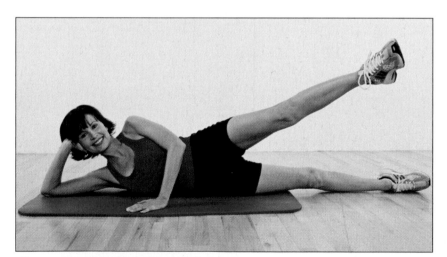 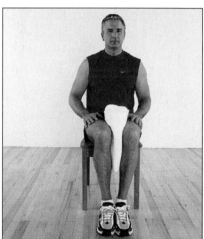

3. Side Thrust Kick

From hands and knees to your side for this interesting and challenging move for your hips. **Level 3, page 63**

4. Towel Squeeze

Back up into a chair for this simple isometric exercise for stronger leg muscles that again aid your hips. **Level 1, page 58**

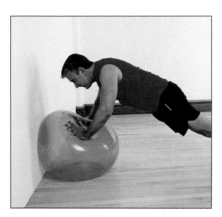

5. Ball Push-Up

Grab the exercise ball again and down on the floor for this challenging chest workout that also tests your balance. **Level 3, page 93**

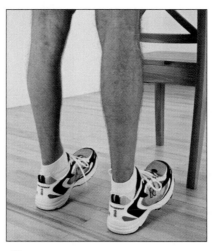

6. Heel/Toe Raise

Great for your feet and ankles, but also for your calf muscles. **Level 2, page 101**

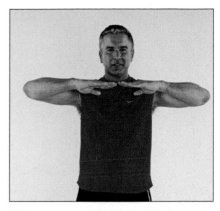

7. Upright Row

This shoulder exercise also forces a good-sized stretch of your elbow joint. **Level 2, page 73**

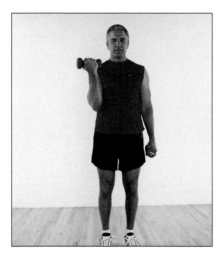

8. Standing Biceps Curl

This classic exercise is not only for good-looking arms but also elbow relief and extra calorie burn. **Level 2, page 108**

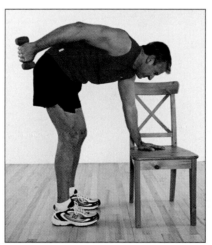

9. Triceps Kickback

Muscle pairs need balance, and so for every biceps exercise you do, you need a triceps exercise. **Level 2, page 107**

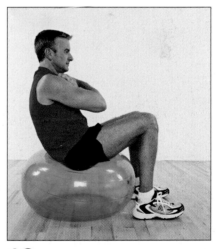

10. Ball Curl

One more time with your exercise ball. This exercise strengthens your abdominal muscles and truly tests your balance. **Level 3, page 81**

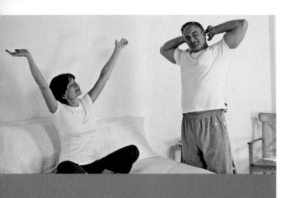

making the Program Work

Each of the three programs uses a different set of exercises and stretches. If you find some to be too easy or difficult, look at exercises prescribed for the same area of the body in the next level up or down. But if possible, try to follow the program as outlined. What to do when the workout gets too easy? Follow the progression guidelines outlined in the Total Body Stretch and Total Body Strength programs. Boiled down, they say to start with a low number of repetitions and build toward higher repetitions and multiple sets as you become stronger. These programs should take under 30 minutes.

Aside from pain, the most devastating consequence of arthritis is its ability to rob you of movement and prevent you from going

about normal daily activities. These programs build strength and range of motion in all the body's major joints and muscle groups, but focus especially on large muscles that are important for gross motor functions such as walking, climbing stairs, lifting, and doing household chores.

Instructions

Again, we have provided beginning, intermediate, and advanced programs. For each program, there are two main sequences: strengthening and stretching. Here is how to proceed:

> Do a five-minute warmup to get blood flowing throughout your body. Walking in place will do just fine.

> Proceed with the strength exercises. Beginners should start with one set of 6 repetitions for each exercise; intermediate, one set of 6 to 8 repetitions; and advanced, one set of 8 repetitions.

> Next, shift to the flexibility exercises.

> **BEGINNING** Strength Program

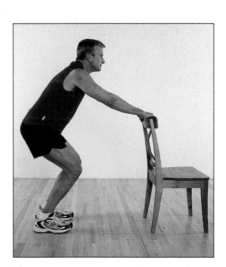

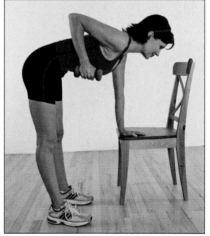

1. **Partial Squat**

Start your program by lengthening thigh muscles that support both hips and knees. **Level 1 or 2, page 57**

2. **Bent Single Arm Row**

This deceptively challenging exercise is for your back, not your arms! No weights makes it easier. **Level 1 or 2, page 88**

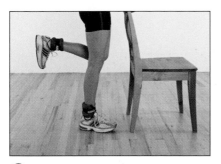

3. Standing Knee Flexion

A simple but effective exercise for your knees and hips. **Level 2, page 60**

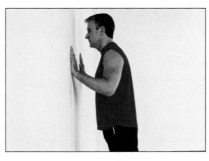

4. Wall Push-Up

This modified version of the classic military exercise gently challenges your chest muscles. **Level 1, page 91**

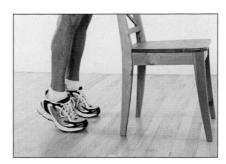

5. Heel Raise

A simple but effective workout for your ankles and feet. Do it anywhere, anytime. **Level 1, page 100**

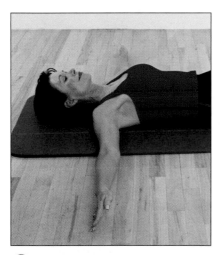

6. Lying Lateral Raise

Down on your back, slowly and carefully, to do this wonderful shoulder workout. **Level 1, page 71**

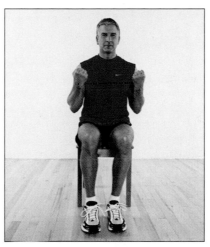

7. Seated Biceps Curl

Up into a chair so you can do this classic elbow-enhancing exercise. **Level 1, page 105**

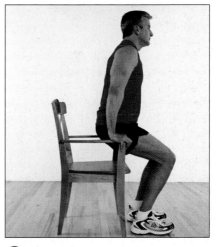

8. Armchair Dip

Carefully lower and raise yourself for arm strength and elbow support. **Level 1, page 106**

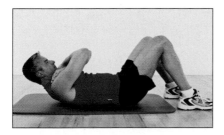

9. Basic or Advanced Abdominal Curl

End your strengthening sequence with this classic stomach test, and turn the page for your flexibility routine! **Level 2 or 3, page 78 or 80**

> **BEGINNING** Flexibility Program

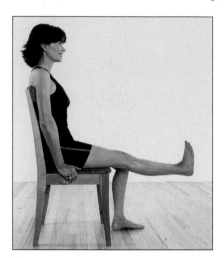

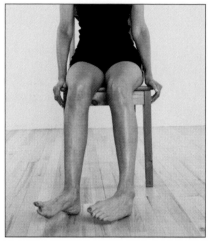

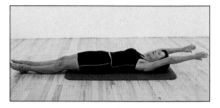

1. Seated Knee Extension

Gentle and easy, but hold it for best effect. Add weights to your ankle and you have a wonderful leg-strengthening exercise. **Page 52**

2. Ankle Circle

Again, gentle and easy, but surprisingly refreshing for your feet. Walk around and you'll see. **Page 98**

3. Lying Total Body Stretch

The most natural of movements—you see wild animals do it all the time—and for good reason: it refreshes and rejuvenates. **Page 77**

everyday *secrets*

THE GROCERIES

Sometimes hard on joints but also hard to avoid, grocery shopping—with its reaching, grasping, lifting, hauling, loading, and putting away—can be a challenging chore when you have arthritis. To make the job easier:

Bolster your bags. Why struggle wrestling groceries in paper bags without handles or plastic bags that pinch your hands under heavy loads? Alternative: Bring your own cloth bags with thick handles made of canvas or wooden dowels (sometimes provided by libraries, offered as premiums from charities such as public broadcasting, or available from catalogs such as L. L. Bean). Tell the checkout clerk how heavy you want the bags: When the weight is comfortable for your hands, carrying will work the muscles of your shoulders, arms, and back. Start with light loads and add an extra item each time you go to the supermarket.

Walk the aisles. Don't aimlessly wander the grocery aisles—purposely make it a goal to stroll down every one of them, whether you need to pick something off the shelves or not. You'll build extra steps of walking into your day and may actually remember to pick up the paprika you ran out of last week. If browsing along the way makes it too tempting to pick up food you don't need, stick to the perimeter of the store (where healthy foods like fresh produce tend to be) or circulate through aisles you've already shopped.

Unload piecemeal. When you get home with your groceries, avoid loading yourself down with multiple bags. Instead, get one bag from the car at a time, which prevents pain from stressing arthritic joints while building strength and adding to your daily accumulation of steps.

Bag it yourself. First, the exercise is good for you. Second, you can organize your bags for easier unloading when at home. And third, you'll win friends by helping speed up the checkout line, since fewer and fewer grocery stores have baggers. ■

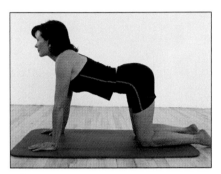

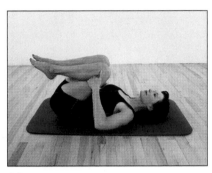

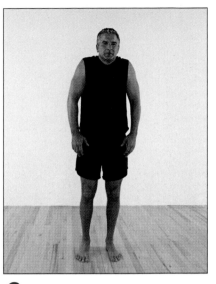

4. Cat Stretch

A little more strenuous, but again, very natural and wonderful for your back. **Page 84**

5. Knees to Chest

Chances are you spent many hours of your childhood in this position. Stretch your back again and regain your youthful spirit. **Page 55**

6. Shoulder Roll

When your neck or upper back aches, you do this move naturally for relief. Do it now for flexibility and shoulder relief. **Page 68**

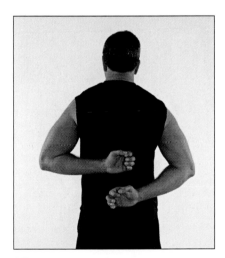

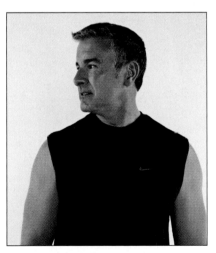

7. Knuckle Rub

At first, this seems difficult. But in time, you will find your knuckles will rise farther up your back as your body grows more flexible. **Page 69**

8. Neck Turn

End this routine with yet another movement we do naturally to re-lieve tension and provide soothing relief. **Page 94**

> INTERMEDIATE Strength Program

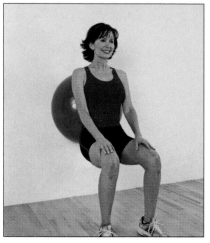

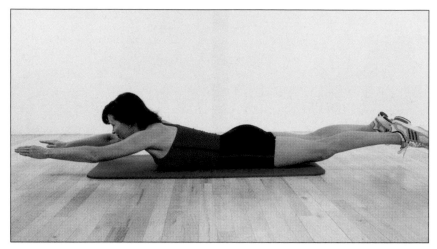

1. Ball Squat

This is challenging in two ways: Squats truly test your leg muscles, and balancing the large ball takes practice. But the benefits are great! **Level 3, page 63**

2. Superman

You'd think this would be an arm and leg exercise, but it is the muscles in your torso that provide the lift and balance. **Level 2, page 87**

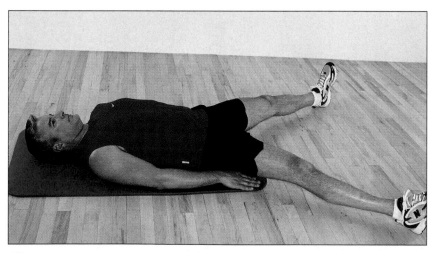

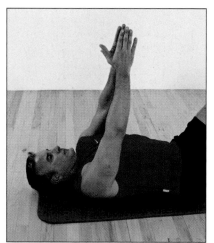

3. Lying Hip Abduction

No need to try doing a full split! Gently open your legs until you feel tension, and stop. In time, you will be able to widen the split. **Level 1, page 57**

4. Chest Fly

This seems natural and easy, but the weight of your arms makes for a surprisingly good workout. **Level 1, page 92**

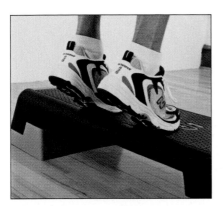

5. Stair Heel Raise

While you will feel the muscle tension in your calf muscles, this is a very beneficial exercise for your ankles and feet. **Level 2, page 100**

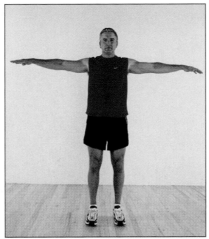

6. Around the World

Next, this shoulder exercise will help you reach more assuredly for things above your head. **Level 2, page 74**

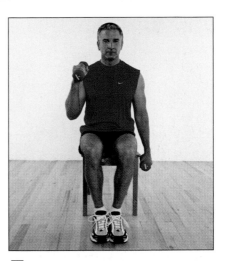

7. Hammer Curl

This variation of the classic biceps curl will provide much relief to your elbow joint. **Level 2, page 107**

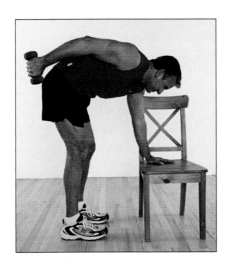

8. Triceps Kickback

Be prepared to feel the tension and fatigue in this upper-arm muscle, which often goes unexercised. **Level 2, page 107**

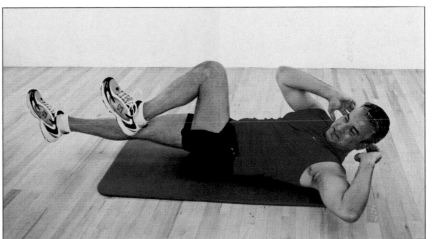

9. Basic or Advanced Bicycle

Great for your abdomen, great for your legs, and even great for your heart and lungs. **Level 2 or 3 depending on variation, page 79 or 81**

> INTERMEDIATE Flexibility Program

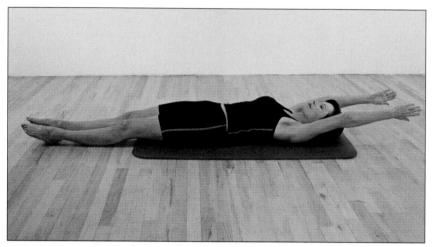

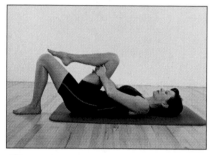

1. Lying Total Body Stretch

We recommend this stretch often because it feels so good, so natural, and so relieving. **Page 77**

2. Low Back Knees to Chest

Don't worry if at first you have a hard time with this move. In time, you'll feel comfortable on your back and with your knees pulled to you. **Page 82**

---

everyday *secrets*

YOUR DAILY DOINGS

As you move throughout your day, you'll benefit from knowing a number of basic skills or tools such as these:

Practice perfect lifts. Doing your workout isn't the only time good form is important. Household tasks are exercise too—and it's just as important to perform everyday movements properly to keep from straining joints and muscles. Lifting objects such as laundry baskets or stacks of newspapers can be particularly hard on the back. But done correctly, lifting can also provide a good workout for muscles and joints. Here's how:

• Get close to the object and try to keep it near your center of gravity, which makes it easier to lift and is less likely to strain your back.

• Keep your back straight and bend at the knees to raise the object off the ground. Avoid bending at the waist and trying to muscle something up using just your back. (If you have knee problems, don't be afraid to ask for help.)

• Once you've completed the lift, don't turn at the waist, but keep the object close to your body, point your toes where you want to go, and turn your entire body.

Stand without strain. When standing for prolonged periods (for example, at the kitchen counter washing dishes or preparing food), take pressure off the lower back by resting one foot on a platform

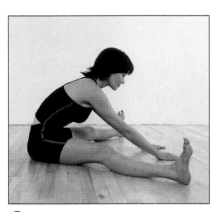

3. Seated V

Another great stretch that seems awkward at first, but becomes natural with just a little practice. **Page 53**

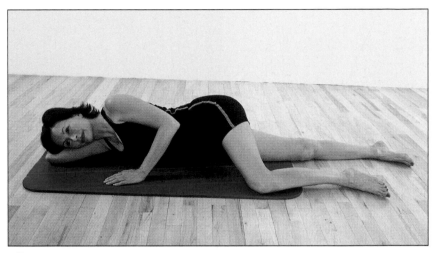

4. Lying Pelvis Rotation

While still on the ground, get on your side and do this gentle stretch for the muscles along the outside of the thigh. **Page 55**

Program continues >

about two to four inches high—about the height of a phone book—and occasionally shifting weight from one foot to another. To fight fatigue while standing, do what you'd think would make you more tired: exercise. Heel raises squeeze your veins, prevent blood from pooling in your extremities, and force blood back to your heart, which actually makes it less tiring to stand for a long time.

Take care on stairs. Going up and down stairs can be a major ordeal for people with arthritis, but

going about it the right way can minimize pain or help prevent it from getting worse. Some ways to do it:

• Although the first priority is to do what's most comfortable, avoid taking steps one foot at a time, leading with the better foot. Constantly favoring one foot generally causes one side to become stronger than the other, making problems worse, not better. A better way: If it's safe to do so, take steps evenly using both feet, using the rail for support.

• Use your arms for support and balance, but don't use them to lift yourself up the stairs, which can lead to pain in the shoulders.

• Be particularly dedicated to exercises for the quadriceps muscles of the thighs, which are primary movers both for going up stairs and the more difficult braking action of going down.

Use a cane. Some people with arthritis feel using a cane makes them seem old or crippled, but it's

continued on page 154

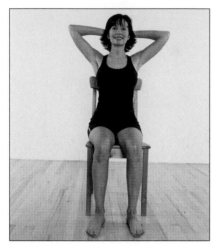

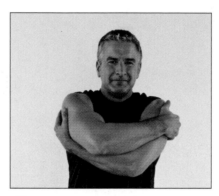

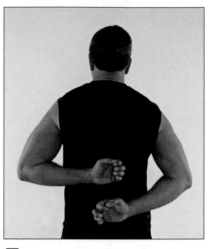

5. Seated Chest Stretch

Now get up and sit in a chair to give the muscles in the front of your shoulders and the top of your chest a good stretch. **Page 90**

6. Self-Hug

This is among the most simple and intuitive of stretches. Yet it really does aid your shoulders for greater mobility. **Page 68**

7. Knuckle Rub

A less natural movement, but also quite good for a different set of shoulder muscles. **Page 69**

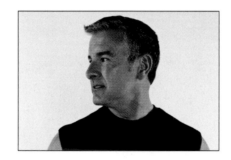

8. Neck Turn

Finish this routine with stretches for those often stressed and tense neck muscles. **Page 94**

continued from page 153

better to think of it strictly as a functional tool that takes pressure off the hips. Ways to link "cane" and "able":

• Hold the cane in the hand opposite the side that hurts, which studies find reduces the load on the hip by 50 percent. Using a cane on the wrong side actually increases pressure on the hip.

• Be sure the length of the cane matches your height, ideally coming about wrist high when your arm is hanging at your side. A cane that's longer than that stresses the arm, and a cane that's shorter makes you lean, which puts pressure on the back.

• If you don't want a cane to look like a medical piece, go for style. Some canes are carved from tree branches and lacquered; others are painted with vines and birds.

• Canes aren't designed to bear your weight, but if you want hip (as in "cool") support and stability from something other than a cane, consider walking with the help of trekking poles made of high-tech materials such as titanium. ■

> ADVANCED Strength Program

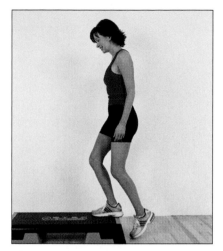

1. Stair Step-Up

For greater mobility, nothing is more practical than exercising the muscles used to climb stairs or hills. **Level 2 or 3 depending on variation, page 61**

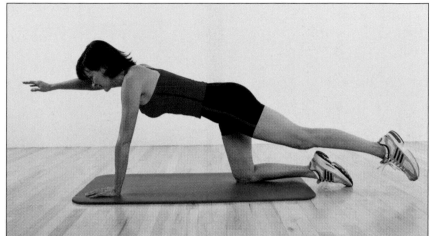

2. Bird Dog

This exercise strengthens your back for easier stretching and reaching. **Level 2, page 62**

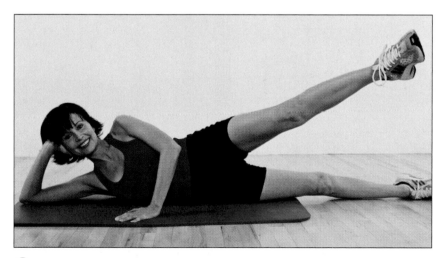

3. Side Thrust Kick

While this does not feel natural at first, it will build important muscles and become easy before you know it. **Level 3, page 63**

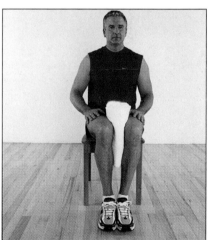

4. Towel Squeeze

Amazing how much beneficial strengthening you can do merely by squeezing your legs together in this way. **Level 1, page 58**

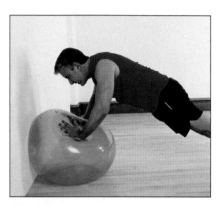

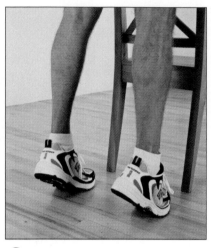

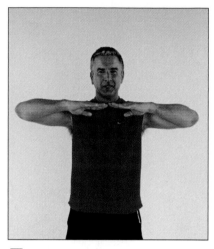

5. Ball Push-Up

This exercise is great for hands, arms, chest, and overall balance and strength. **Level 3, page 93**

6. Heel/Toe Raise

While it is the calf muscles that get tested the most, this exercise is great for all parts of your feet. **Level 2, page 101**

7. Upright Row

Strong chest muscles make all your lifting and throwing much, much easier to do. **Level 2, page 73**

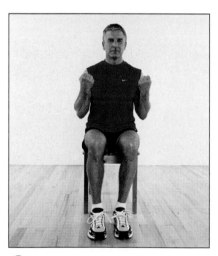

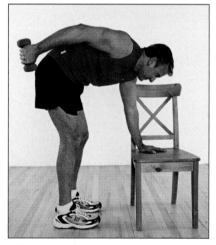

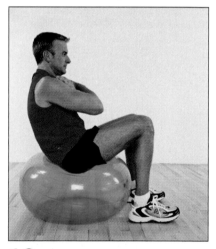

8. Seated Biceps Curl

Strong biceps will make lifting and carrying things much easier as well. **Level 2, page 105**

9. Triceps Kickback

Muscle pairs, like the biceps and triceps, need to be balanced, so don't neglect the less showy muscle opposite your biceps. **Level 2, page 107**

10. Ball Curl

End this mobility-strength program with an abdomen exercise that has a sense of fun and excitement. Don't fall off the ball! **Level 3, page 81**

> **ADVANCED** Flexibility Program

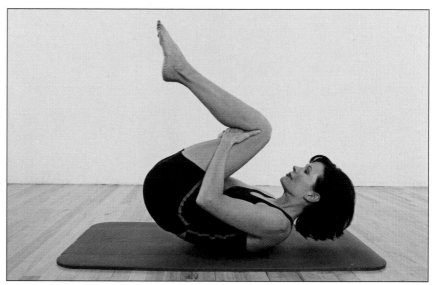

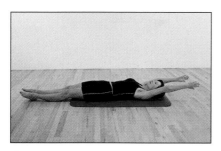

1. Lying Total Body Stretch

For optimal mobility, you want your entire body to be loose and flexible. This opening stretch gets you on your way. **Page 77**

2. Rocking Chair

At first, it might feel awkward to curl up on your back like this. But this stretch is soothing and effective. Do it on a carpet or mat for comfort. **Page 83**

Program continues >

everyday *secrets*

WORKING OUTSIDE

Just about any chore outdoors involves major joints and muscles important for mobility—which can make yard and garden tasks especially challenging. But the physical labor is good for your muscles, so it's worth doing all you can, with steps like the following to ease discomfort.

Fashion hefty handles. When using lawn and garden tools such as rakes and hoes, make the handles easier to grasp the way hockey players wearing mitts do: Wrap the handle in athletic tape to make it thicker—and wear gloves when working to protect sensitive hands.

Don't work too hard in the yard. Take a break every 15 minutes when gardening. It's easy to become engrossed in yard work, but while the labor counts as exercise, you want to avoid getting too much of a good thing, lest you overwork your abdomen and lower back. Frequent rests help your muscles relax and make the work more pleasant. In addition, switch sides frequently to avoid overworking a single muscle group—and use exercises such as the bicycle to get your torso into shape.

continued on page 158

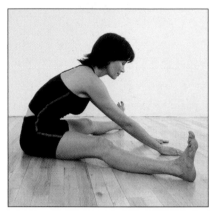

3. Seated V

Now into a seated position with legs straight out. This stretch is great for your hips and challenges your whole body. **Page 53**

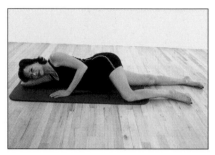

4. Lying Pelvis Rotation

Lie down on your back and get those legs rolling above you. Outstanding for your hips, and a general feel-good move as well. **Page 55**

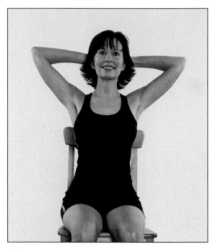

5. Seated Chest Stretch

Back up to a chair—or even standing, if you like—to stretch the often-tense muscles at the top of your chest and the front of your shoulders. **Page 90**

continued from page 157

Give yourself a raise. Planting a garden doesn't have to take place at ground level. Instead of stooping to the dirt, use raised beds so you can exercise your green thumb from a seated or standing position.

Take a seat. Kneeling for planting or weeding can be hard on knees. A better position: Sitting low to the ground on a bucket, stool, or small wagon. Check gardening centers, catalogs, or websites for garden carts that can be loaded and pulled, but close with a lid that doubles as a seat. Alternative position: Try lying on your hip or side for tasks such as hand digging or weeding.

Cushion your knees. If you need to kneel and your joints comfortably allow it, use pads made of closed-cell foam, which cushions without compressing flat. You can order knee pads and other "enabling" tools for the garden from specialized Internet websites such as gardenscapetools.com.

Take the rigor from raking. When using a rake, take shorter strokes instead of reaching out away from the body, which puts more stress on joints, especially the back. Bend your knees slightly when stroking, to allow muscles of the legs and hips to contribute more to the motion. Plus, this posture eases strain on the upper body

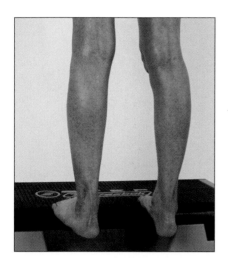

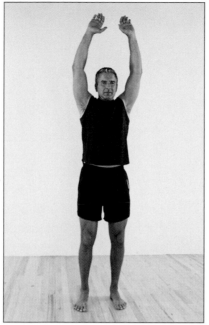

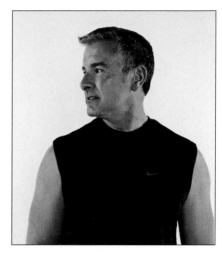

6. Stair Calf Stretch

Chances are you'll "feel the burn" in your calves as you do this classic stretch for your lower legs and ankles. **Page 98**

7. "Good Morning" Exercise

Wonderful for your shoulders. Feel your rib cage spread and take in some deep breaths to refresh your whole body. **Page 70**

8. Neck Turn

The classic way to end a stretching routine. Tension often lands in your neck, so let it release. **Page 94**

and protects your back.

Throw in the trowel. Digging with a trowel can be tough on arthritic hands. To make it easier, start with the narrowest implement you can find: Tools with wider blades create more resistance in the dirt. When digging, chop with the trowel to loosen clumped dirt, then insert the trowel no deeper than half its length to loosen the soil and avoid straining against more densely packed deeper layers. Work your way deeper with short scoops.

Be sure with a shovel. As with a trowel, you want to dig with a shovel in shallow bits, gradually loosening dirt in small shovelfuls. Use your legs to lift the dirt, doing a partial squat to gain leverage, keeping hands close to your body to avoid stressing your back. Avoid placing the shovel too far in front of you. Instead, keep the load within a couple of feet to promote better posture and balance as you work. If you place the shovel farther than that, lunge forward with one knee to keep your body's center of gravity close to the load.

Work standing up. When planting seeds, sharpen one end of a broomstick to make holes in the soil, then drop seeds from a standing position using a long piece of small-diameter PVC piping cut to about waist height. ■

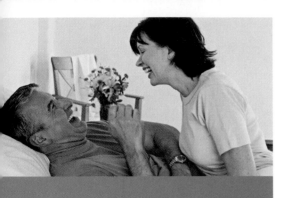

making the
Program Work

These programs consist entirely of upper-body exercises and stretches. Progress in the order indicated, starting with large muscles that support the extremities and working toward finer movements of the hands and wrists. Follow the progression guidelines outlined in the Total Body Stretch and Total Body Strength programs, beginning strength programs with the starting number of sets and repetitions indicated.

Dexterity usually refers to fine motor control—the ability to write, draw, cook, pick up objects with your fingers, and work with tools

or crafts. But you need more than nimble fingers to use hands effectively; you also need strong and supple muscles in the upper body, especially around the shoulders, upper back, front of the chest, and arms. Stabilizing this area, known as the shoulder girdle, provides greater control, endurance, and overall function of your extremities, allowing more refined movements in the hands and wrists.

Instructions

We've provided beginning, intermediate, and advanced programs. For each program, there are two main sequences: strengthening and stretching. Here is how to proceed:

> Do a five-minute warmup to get blood flowing throughout your body. Walking in place will do just fine, though since this is an upper-body program, be sure your arms have participated in the warmup.

> Proceed with the strength exercises. Beginners should start with one set of 6 repetitions for each exercise; intermediate, one set of 6 to 8 repetitions; and advanced, one set of 8 repetitions.

> Next, shift to the flexibility exercises.

> BEGINNING Strength Program

Starting point: 1 set of 6 repetitions

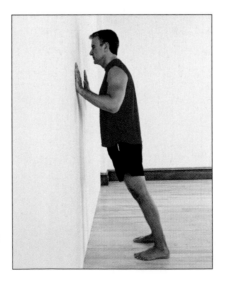

1. Wall Push-Up

This standing version of the classic floor push-up still gives your chest and arms a good workout. **Level 1, page 91**

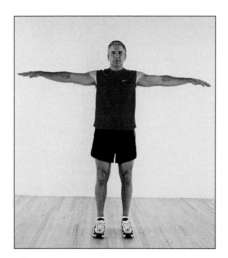

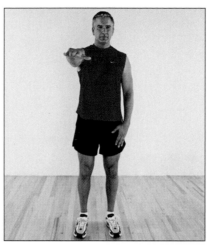

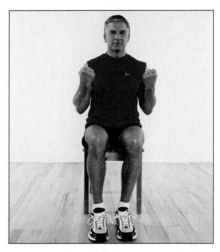

2. Standing Lateral Raise

Use the weight of your arms to build up shoulder and neck muscles. **Level 2, page 73**

3. Front Raise

Similar to lateral raises, but this exercise strengthens a different set of shoulder and back muscles. **Level 2, page 74**

4. Seated Biceps Curl

You may not think that strong upper arms will help your dexterity, but they offer key support to your elbows and shoulders. **Level 1, page 105**

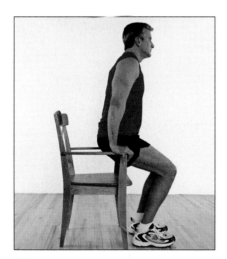

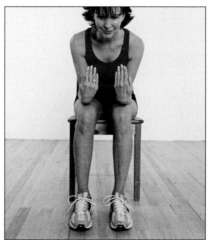

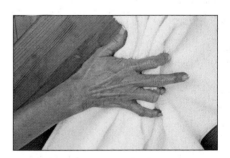

5. Armchair Dip

While the main muscles strengthened here are in your arms, this everyday movement is great for overall dexterity and motion. **Level 1, page 106**

6. Wrist Curl

Now to the muscles of the wrist and forearm. Though smaller in size than the upper-arm muscles, they need strengthening too. **Level 1, page 112**

7. Towel Grab

End this routine with a simple exercise for stronger fingers and hands. **All levels, page 117**

> **BEGINNING** Flexibility Program

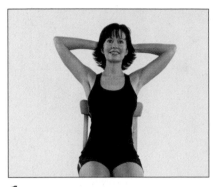

1. Seated Chest Stretch

Use the weight of your arms to provide your chest muscles a long, full stretch. **Page 90**

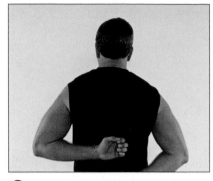

2. Knuckle Rub

Now stretch your upper arms and shoulder joint by carefully gliding your knuckles along your spine. **Page 69**

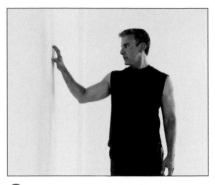

3. Wall Climb

Don't be self-conscious doing this stretch, and don't rush through it. It is particularly good for people with limited dexterity. **Page 69**

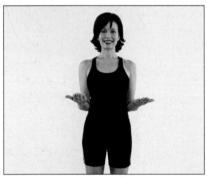

4. Forearm Flip

This both stretches and strengthens the muscles in your forearm, making elbow and wrist movement easier. **Page 104**

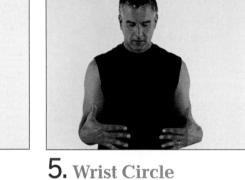

5. Wrist Circle

A relatively small movement, but wrist stretches like these can make all the difference in your everyday functioning. **Page 111**

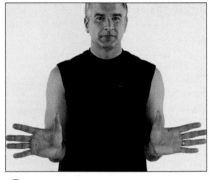

6. Handshake Wrist Bend

Another wrist stretch that uses a different motion to help your manual dexterity. **Page 110**

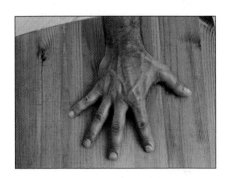

7. Finger Stretch

Don't think that because you use fingers all day, they don't need strengthening and stretching. This flex does wonders! **Page 116**

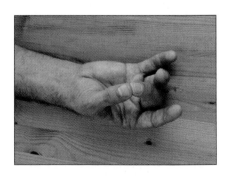

8. Thumb Touch

Finally, end your dexterity workout with this simple sequence for your hands and fingers. **Page 116**

> INTERMEDIATE Strength Program

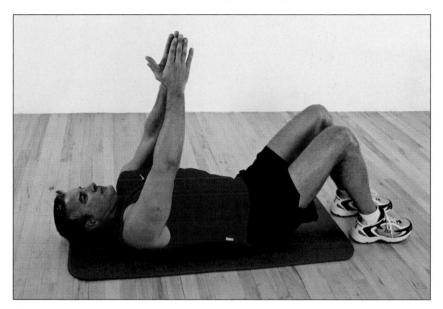

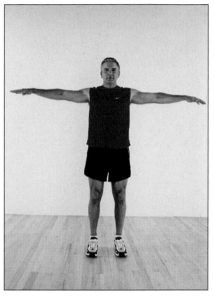

1. Chest Fly

Lying on your back, you are strengthening your chest, arms, and shoulders with this unweighted arm lift. **Level 1, page 92**

2. Around the World

Now back on your feet to move your arms from another perspective, giving them a full range of motion as well as more strength. **Level 2, page 74**

Program continues >

---

everyday *secrets*

Clothing

When fingers and wrists ache, when bending and pulling are a challenge, getting dressed can become an ordeal. While exercises and stretches can improve your ability to dress easily, you can also take steps to make the routine easier:

Buy big. Instead of buying clothes—especially shirts, blouses, jackets, and sweatshirts—with perfect fit in mind, choose items that are a size too big through the body or made with a roomy cut, to give you extra room when wrestling them on and off. Avoid items that lack "give," such as denim and tweed, or are difficult to get over your head, such as turtlenecks.

Cut demands on hands. Choose pants with elastic waists that are easy to pull on and off, sparing your hands painful manipulation of buttons or zippers. When you can't avoid the use of fasteners, choose items such as skirts, dresses, shirts, blouses, and bras that zip or fasten on the side or front instead the back. If you're stuck with difficult-to-reach fasteners, try positioning the garment so you can reach a zipper, button, or clasp in front, then move the item into proper position. When possible, use fasteners made with Velcro or large, flat buttons that are easy to handle.

Reorganize your closet. An organized closet doesn't just look better—it might make you feel better. Instead of heaping shoes

continued on page 164

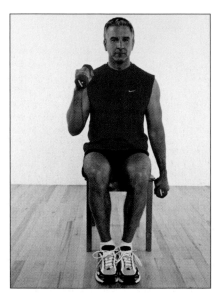

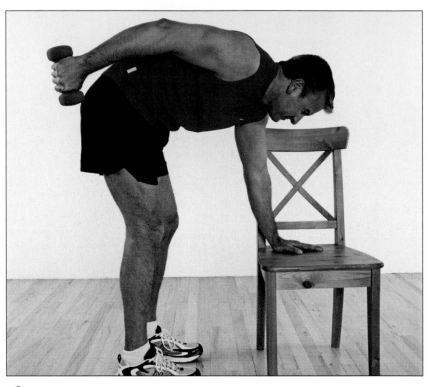

3. Hammer Curl

This seated curl strengthens forearm muscles that help support your elbow, working on a different part of the arm from biceps curls. **Level 2, page 107**

4. Triceps Kickback

Use an armless chair or a bench for this exercise that works on the muscles at the bottom of your upper arm. **Level 2, page 107**

---

continued from page 163

on the floor of your closet—where you have to bend and sort them—get a hanging shoe rack for a wall or door so footwear is within easy reach. And if reaching for hangers at or above shoulder height is difficult, lower the bar of your hanging rack. Meantime, take items off the rack using two hands, or grasping items between a hand and your arm or wrist.

Prepare for morning. If you know you're going to feel stiff in the morning, lay out clothes the night

before, when it's easier to search through closets, paw through drawers, and handle the items you choose.

Be deliberate with drawers. Most dressers come with bottom drawers that are larger and tough to open. Though it's natural to organize drawers by content size, with bulky things in bigger drawers, think instead in terms of how often clothes are used, putting frequently worn items in smaller drawers closer to the top, where they're easier to reach and handle.

Sit to stand. To make putting on pants easier (and to make sure pain while dressing doesn't cause you to lose your balance), sit down on the edge of a bed or chair to pull trousers over your legs, then stand up to hitch the waist.

Do the splits. They're popular with kids, but immensely useful for people with arthritis—pants with zippers in the legs that can turn a pair of long trousers into shorts without taking the entire garment off and replacing it with another. You can get them at stores catering to young shoppers, but a better bet

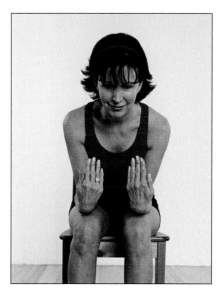

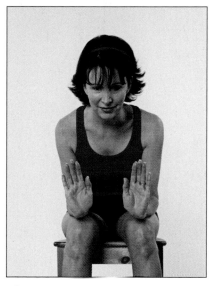

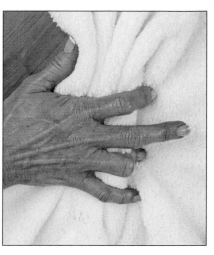

5. Wrist Curl

Back in a chair, you can now start toning up muscles closer to your hands—those of your wrists—that support your hands as they tackle jobs like piano playing or sewing.
Level 1, page 118

6. Wrist Extension

Here you are working on the muscles opposite the ones you put to use in the wrist curls, a balance that helps both sets of muscles.
Level 1, page 118

7. Towel Grab

A seemingly silly exercise that a pet cat might think was a game for its pleasure is designed to help rebuild dexterity in stiff fingers.
All levels, page 117

may be sporting goods stores or catalogs, which often feature light-weight convertible clothes for hiking and multi-sport activities.

Use donning devices. You'll find it easier to get into a variety of garments with special devices designed to help with manipulation. (Check a medical supply store or Internet websites such as aids-forarthritis.com or independent-needs.com.) Devices include:

• buttonhooks, featuring a handle holding a wire that grasps buttons and pulls them through buttonholes

• sock aids, in which a shell holds the sock in place as you slip your foot into it, and allows you to pull it up using long handles

• long shoehorns with extended handles that allow you to get feet into shoes without bending over

• zipper pullers, which grab zippers with a hook and allow you to slide them with the help of a handle

Focus on footwear. Getting shoes on is half the battle. The other half is getting them to stay. Laces can be hard on arthritic fingers, but if they're made of elastic, you

need only tie shoes once and they'll stay snapped tight until you want your shoes off. Some stylish shoes now on the market come already laced with knot-free elastic cord: You just slip the shoes on and off without tying anything—the elastic conforms to your foot. Other options include shoes that close with Velcro. ■

> **INTERMEDIATE** Flexibility Program

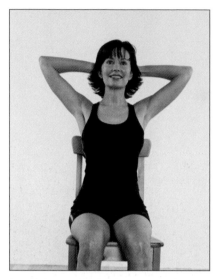

1. Seated Chest Stretch

You can sit or stand while you try to lengthen the muscles of your upper chest and the front of your shoulders; as you repeat, your arms will go further back. **Page 90**

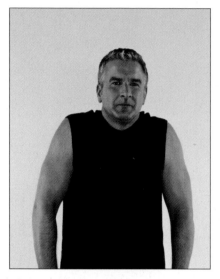

2. Shoulder Roll

A good stretch for your shoulders, this is also a relaxing exercise for tense shoulder and neck muscles. **Page 68**

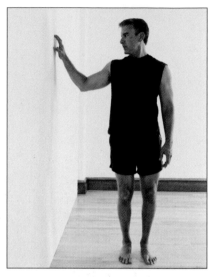

3. Wall Climb

Working out both your shoulders and your fingers, this exercise helps increase your shoulder muscles' range of motion. **Page 69**

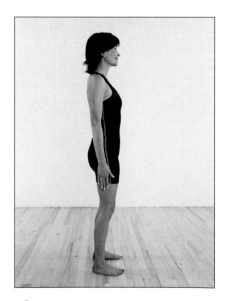

4. Arm Hang

For elbows that are stiff and bent, this stretch helps you gradually straighten your arm all the way again. **Page 104**

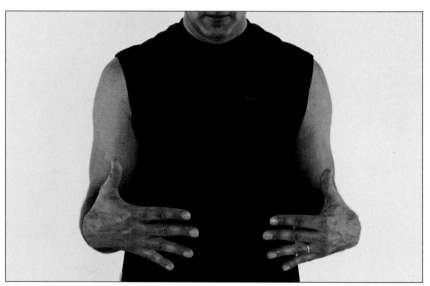

5. Wrist Circle

This simple stretch, which seems like drawing circles in the air, incorporates all the movements of the wrist in a continuous motion. **Page 111**

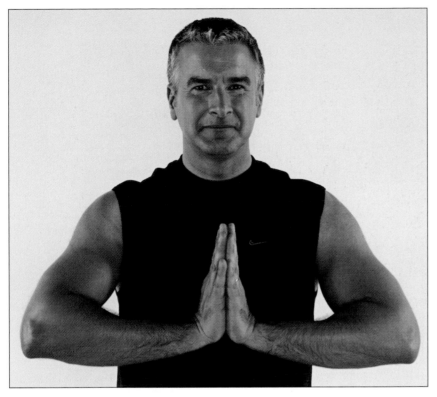

6. Prayer Stretch

This pious-looking stretch lengthens muscles in your elbows, forearms, and wrists. **Page 111**

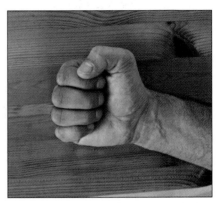

7. Gentle Fist

The movements of this stretch give your fingers a relaxing work-out while also expanding their range of motion. **Page 116**

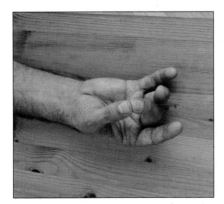

8. Thumb Touch

Finger dexterity depends on the movements of this stretch, which involves each finger individually. And remember: You can do this anytime! **Page 116**

> **ADVANCED** Strength Program Starting point: 1 set of 8 repetitions.

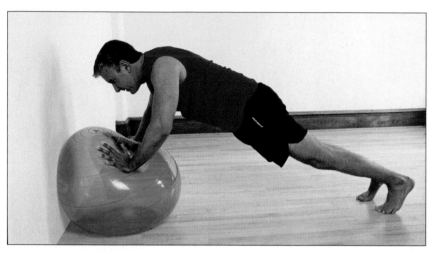

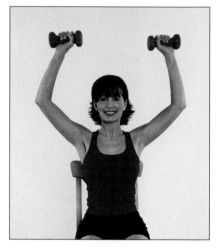

1. Ball Push-Up

Now you're working out the larger muscles that support your arms and hands in a strength exercise that also requires balance. **Level 3, page 93**

2. Overhead Dumbbell Press

Onto an armless chair or bench for this classic exercise that strengthens your shoulders, upper back, and upper arms. **Level 3, page 75**

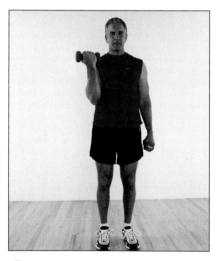

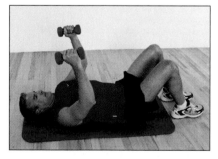

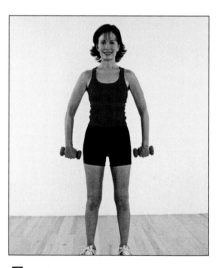

3. Standing Biceps Curl

Stand up for this set of curls—it works muscles in your torso and lower body as well as your shoulder and arms because it requires some balance. **Level 3, page 108**

4. Lying Triceps Extension

Back on the mat for more shoulder and arm work, giving a strong base to your wrists and hands. **Level 3, page 109**

5. Standing Wrist Curl

There is a twist to these curls that affects muscles in your forearms not touched by other curls. **Level 3, page 115**

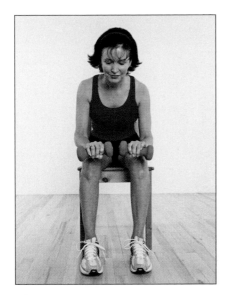

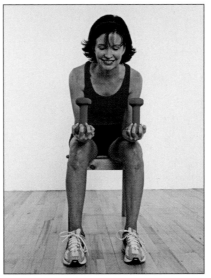

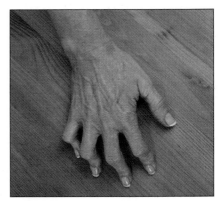

6. Weighted Wrist Extension

Sit down for this exercise, which strengthens the muscles of your wrists with repetition, then greater weights. **Level 2, page 114**

7. Thor's Hammer

Still in your chair, grab the weights by their ends for this rotation exercise that also strengthens your wrists. **Level 3, page 115**

8. Spider Walk

Fingers are the beneficiaries of this tabletop exercise that can be done with all fingers at once or with individual ones as you get stronger. **All levels, page 117**

everyday *secrets*

In the Kitchen

Cooking is not only a necessity but, for many of us, a pleasure. Here are ways to make the process easier when arthritis challenges your dexterity:

Leverage lids. You can use an electric can opener to take the tops off most cans, but pop-top cans for products such as soft drinks, pet food, nuts, or canned frosting often lack the metal lip that an opener requires to work. Options: Use a knife to pry the top off a soda pop can or use the handle of a spoon as a lever to take off a vacuum pack lid. Otherwise, try flipping the can over: The bottom may be the right shape for your can opener. To loosen tight lids on small bottles, reach for a nutcracker: The toothy, gripping gap for the nut is the perfect size for grasping and wrenching bottle caps.

Strain, don't drain. Instead of hefting a pot of boiled food to the sink so you can dump water through a strainer, get a kettle with a perforated insert that holds food but can be lifted out of the water, leaving the heavy pot behind. Have a family member on cleanup duty dump the water later.

Choose the right knife. Cutting with a regular knife may prove difficult when arthritis affects

continued on page 170

> **ADVANCED** Flexibility Program

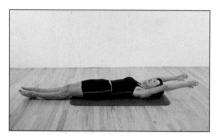

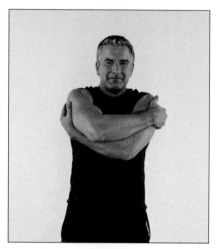

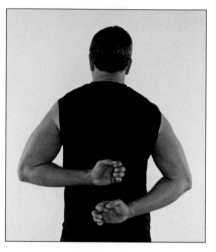

1. Total Body Stretch

Standing or lying in bed, this great stretch gets the kinks out and makes your whole body feel better. **Page 77**

2. Self-Hug

You're not just building self-esteem with this hug; you're stretching muscles in the back of your shoulders. **Page 68**

3. Knuckle Rub

The more you practice this behind-your-back stretch, the farther up your spine you'll be able to go as you stretch the muscles of your shoulders and upper arms. **Page 69**

continued from page 169

hands and wrists, but special L-shaped knives allow you to grip an upright handle that keeps stress off your wrist. In some cases, you can also make what you're cutting easier to deal with: Soaking potatoes in warm water, for example, softens the skin and makes them less challenging to peel.

Arrange for reaching. No kitchen seems to have enough cabinet space, but to make best use of yours, use the lower cupboards for the items you use most frequently, to cut down on the need to reach over your head, putting stress on your shoulder joints. Next priority: Put heavier items on lower shelves and lighter ones up higher. If you find you need to reach overhead often, try using a tool that features a pincher grip on the end of a long handle that can be used to pick up a variety of objects.

Take cups from cupboards. To clear room from cabinets so you can manage their contents more effectively, take frequently used cups out of the cupboard altogether and instead hang them from pegs underneath.

Jump-start juicing. Save yourself effort when using a hand juicer for oranges or grapefruits by rolling the fruit firmly on the counter with your palm before you slice and juice. The pressure will loosen the flesh from the rind and boost your juice output. ■

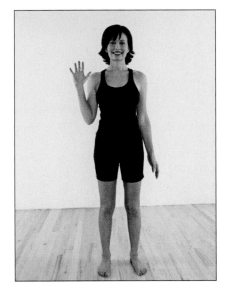

4. Shoulder Touch

Your arms go to your sides for this elbow-bending stretch; keep your elbows close to your waist throughout. **Page 105**

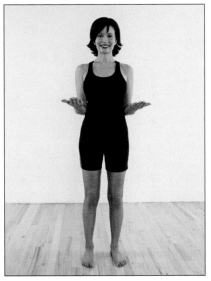

5. Forearm Flip

Here's another elbow stretch that works on range of motion in that often-stiff joint. **Page 104**

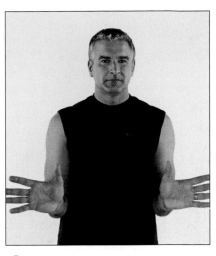

6. Handshake Wrist Bends

Keep your hands moving in this stretch designed primarily for the wrists. **Page 110**

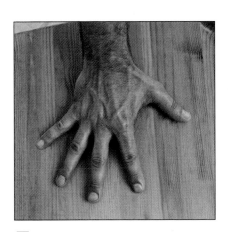

7. Finger Stretch

Separate your fingers as far as you can; then relax and do it again. It will feel great. **Page 116**

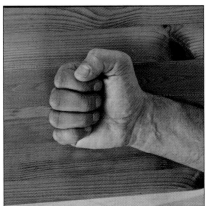

8. Gentle Fist

Slowly curling up and opening stiff joints will help them become more nimble again. **Page 116**

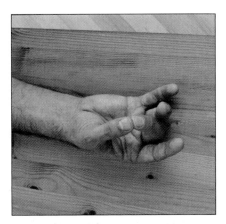

9. Thumb Touch

Here's a good way to check on the mobility of all your fingers and keep them moving at the same time. **Page 116**

Those who play regularly know that golf is a pleasure that is hard to give up. If arthritis is hampering your game, try to make this diverse program of exercise and stretches a three-times-a-week habit. A golf swing is a total body activity that gets much of its power from the lower body and back. The twisting and rotation of each stroke can be hard even on people without arthritis, so you'll need to strengthen and improve mobility of joints and muscles involved with multiple planes of motion, particularly in the hips and spine.

> Strength Exercises

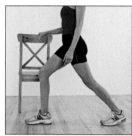

1. Partial Stationary Lunge
Level 3, page 64

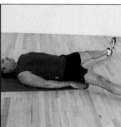

2. Lying Hip Abduction
Level 1, page 57

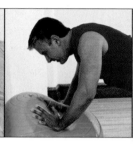

3. Ball Push-Up
Level 3, page 93

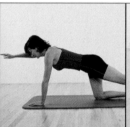

4. Bird Dog
Level 2, page 87

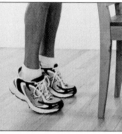

5. Heel Raise
Level 1, page 100

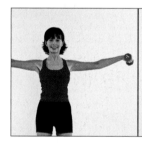

6. Weighted Lateral Raise
Level 3, page 75

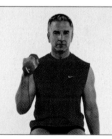

7. Hammer Curl
Level 2, page 107

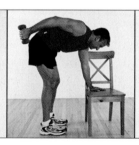

8. Triceps Kickback
Level 2, page 107

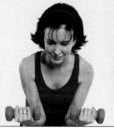

9. Weighted Wrist Curl
Level 2, page 113

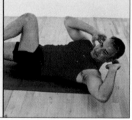

10. Basic or Advanced Bicycle
Level 2 or 3 depending on variation, pages 79 or 81

everyday *secrets*

On the Course

Do a pre-round stretch. Heading to the first tee without first warming up and loosening your joints is a good way to hurt yourself. Take a few minutes before the round begins and do a sequence of stretches that readies your torso for the twisting, your arms for the swinging, your legs for the walking, and your neck and shoulders for the straining.

Consider new grips. Consult with your favorite pro shop or golf store about options for easier-to-handle grips. Regripping a set of clubs with larger, spongier grips may be less costly than you think.

Manage your gear. Tees, ball markers, small pencils, and leather gloves are all a part of the game that can be a challenge for people with arthritis. You can't do without most of them, but you can

Instructions

At least three times a week, get a 20-minute cardio-vascular workout, such as brisk walking or cycling. And at least twice a week, do this program of 10 strengthening exercises and 10 stretches. It seems like a lot, but can be finished in just 20 minutes. Try to do the exercises and stretches in the order given; they progress from large-muscle groups to small, and rotate through different body areas so as not to overly test a single muscle group.

> Flexibility Exercises

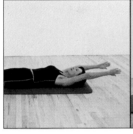 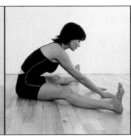 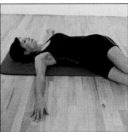 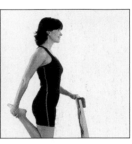

1. Lying Total Body Stretch
Page 77

2. Rocking Chair
Page 83

3. Seated V
Page 53

4. Pelvic Twist
Page 83

5. Standing Quad Stretch
Page 54

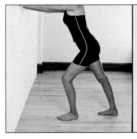 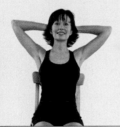 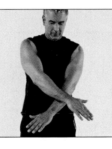 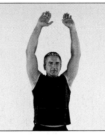 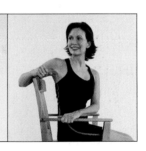

6. Runner's Calf Stretch
Page 99

7. Seated Chest Stretch
Page 90

8. Scissors
Page 70

9. "Good Morning" Exercise
Page 70

10. Seated Torso Twist
Page 76

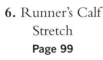

make them easier to access. Try not to keep these things in your pocket, but rather strategically set yourself up, using your bag or your cart for easier access. For example, use a golf glove that has a snap-in ball marker.

Careful with the bending. In golf you are constantly picking up or putting down your ball. It's challenging for your back, neck, and knees. If reaching to the ground over and over proves challenging, squat rather than bend at the waist.

Focus on the abs. When bolstering the torso, don't ignore the abdominal muscles, which support the spine and help power the torso: They're among the most neglected muscles among golfers—perhaps one reason the gut is one of the top areas for golf injuries, even among the pros. ■

[8] Bicycling

Bicycling on a warm, sunny day is one of life's simple pleasures. It is also a wonderful aerobic workout. Even with arthritis, it's a wonderful hobby. Obviously, biking challenges your legs, particularly on hills or long rides. But for many people with arthritis, the real problems lie in the upper body, which tends to fatigue from long periods of supporting much of your body weight on the handlebars.

> Strength Exercises

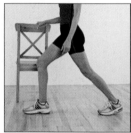

1. Partial Stationary Lunge

Level 3, page 64

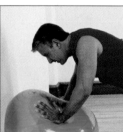

2. Ball Push-Up

Level 3, page 93

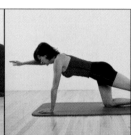

3. Bird Dog

Level 2, page 87

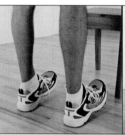

4. Heel/Toe Raise

Level 2, page 101

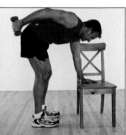

5. Triceps Kickback

Level 2, page 107

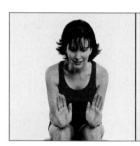

6. Wrist Extension

Level 1, page 112

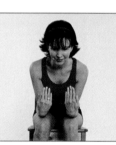

7. Wrist Curl

Level 1, page 112

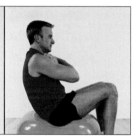

8. Ball Curl

Level 3, page 81

everyday *secrets*

On the Road

Keep the pedals spinning. Stay in a relatively low gear that's easy to pedal, and keep your pedal speed at 80 to 90 revolutions per second (that's about three revolutions every two seconds). That's the secret of the pros, and is smart for you too. Pushing high gears slowly will quickly fatigue your muscles and torture your joints.

Vary your positions. For a seasoned long-distance bicyclist, the goal is to get into one position, one rhythm, and to cover mile after mile. You should be the opposite. To avoid muscle fatigue and aching joints, shift your position constantly. That means moving forward and backward on your seat, holding the handlebars in several different grips, and varying the angle of your back. This variety will ensure you don't

Instructions

This sequence of eight strength exercises and six stretches is custom-made for bicyclists. It emphasizes the key leg muscles, as well as the upper-body strength necessary for a comfortable ride. Do these in sequence three times a week. Start with one set of six reps for the strength exercises, and work up slowly from there. Hold stretches for at least 15 seconds.

> Flexibility Exercises

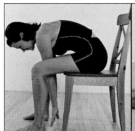 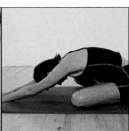 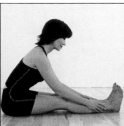 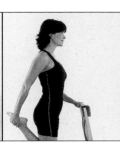 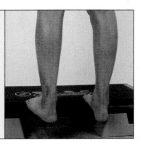

1. Seated Body
Hang
Page 85

2. Cross-Legged
Seated Stretch
Page 84

3. Straight-Leg
Stretch
Page 53

4. Standing Quad
Stretch
Page 54

5. Stair Calf Stretch
Page 98

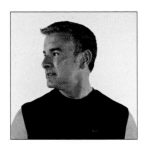

6. Neck Turn
Page 94

overtax a single joint or muscle group.

Rest often. Unless you are in a formal competition, don't compete! This is about fun and health, not speed or distance. Every 15 or 20 minutes, get off the bike and have a rest. Your muscles and joints will appreciate the break—now, and tomorrow when you wake up. And be sure to have enough water on hand to quench your thirst at each break.

Factor in fit. If riding fatigues your upper-body muscles or makes your joints hurt, the problem may be your bike, not your body. Make sure your rig fits you properly by having a bike shop expert size up your frame size and configuration, handlebar position, seat height, and pedal position— all of which count for comfort and mechanical efficiency, especially when you spend long periods in the saddle. ■

[9] Racket Sports

Tennis is a game you just never want to give up. But it is a tough sport on your body (The proof: How many top pros are competitive after the age of 35? Compare that to golf or baseball!) Tennis has many intense physical demands: pivoting, starting and stop- ping, moving quickly in all directions, swinging from all angles. There's not a joint in your body that racket sports don't test. For that reason, people with arthritis who stay with the game need to have a rigorous pro- gram to keep them healthy, fluid, and having fun.

> Strength Exercises

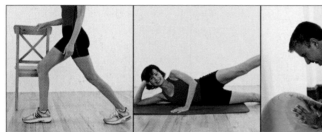
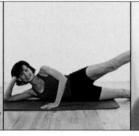
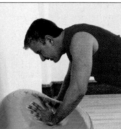
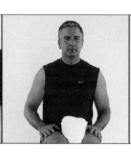
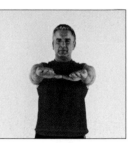

1. Partial Stationary Lunge
Level 3, page 64

2. Side Thrust Kick
Level 3, page 63

3. Ball Push-Up
Level 3, page 93

4. Towel Squeeze
Level 1, page 58

5. Around the World
Level 2, page 74

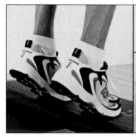
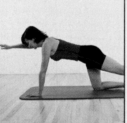
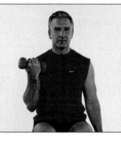
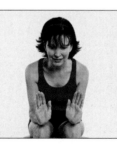
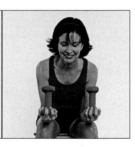

6. Stair Heel Raise
Level 2, page 100

7. Bird Dog
Level 2, page 87

8. Biceps Curl
Level 2, page 106

9. Wrist Extension
Level 1, page 112

10. Thor's Hammer
Level 2, page 115

everyday *secrets*

On the Court

Warm up before starting. Be sure to get your blood flowing and your joints and muscles loosened before starting a game. If not, you greatly increase your chances of joint pain and even injury.

Cushion the impact. It's essential to invest in a good pair of tennis shoes with superior padding to absorb the impact of body weight. Replace your shoes as soon as the heels begin to show wear, be- cause they will no longer be giv- ing you the support you need.

Feet of clay. Clay or Har-Tru courts are much kinder to your joints than hard courts. If you have the choice, always pick clay courts, where the surface absorbs the impact of your steps and you

Instructions

We suggest this three-part workout—aerobic, strengthening, then stretching—three times a week. For the aerobic component, do 20 to 30 minutes of brisk walking. As you become more fit, try to include short bouts (at least 15 seconds at a time) of jogging between 45-second periods of walking, to condition your body to the sport's constant changes of pace. Then do the 10 strength and 10 stretching moves listed here, which should take under 30 minutes. Start the strength exercises with one set of six repetitions. Hold your stretches at least 15 seconds.

> Flexibility Exercises

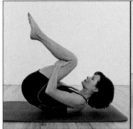
1. Rocking Chair
Page 83

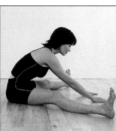
2. Seated V
Page 53

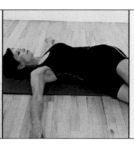
3. Pelvic Twist
Page 83

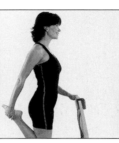
4. Standing Quad Stretch
Page 54

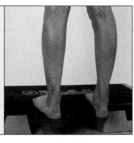
5. Stair Calf Stretch
Page 98

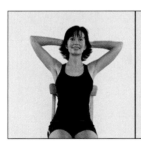
6. Seated Chest Stretch
Page 90

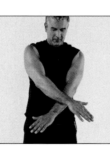
7. Scissors
Page 70

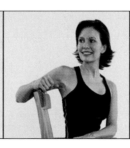
8. Seated Torso Twist
Page 76

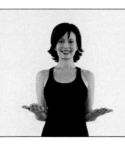
9. Forearm Flip
Page 104

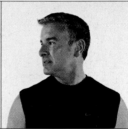
10. Neck Turn
Page 94

can slide into a shot without twisting your ankle.

Double up. Playing doubles is much easier on your knees and ankles because you only have to cover half the court. It also gives you a chance to finally perfect your net game.

The right racket. Modern materials have revolutionized racket design. Most pros will let you test new rackets before you buy and will help you find one that is easier on an arthritic wrist or hand or reverberates less on a stiff elbow.■

Perhaps with the success of a professional league of their own, women will learn what men have long known: Shooting baskets is great fun! And anyone can do it. You can just shoot around, or you can ratchet it up to actually playing games. Shooting is tough on your neck, arms, and shoulders. But the full game of basketball is tough on all of you. In fact, with its sprinting, jumping, pivoting, and twisting, it is among the toughest sports if played full tilt. So if you are serious about maintaining a basketball habit with arthritis, you need a rigorous exercise regimen, like this one.

> Strength Exercises

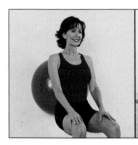 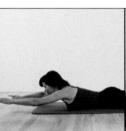 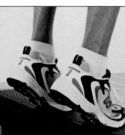 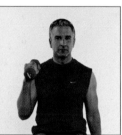 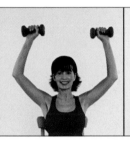

1. Ball Squat
Level 3, page 63

2. Superman
Level 2, page 87

3. Stair Heel Raise
Level 2, page 100

4. Overhead Dumbbell Press
Level 3, page 75

5. Hammer Curl
Level 2, page 107

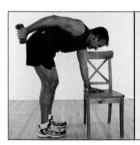 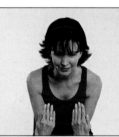 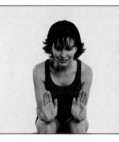 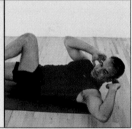

6. Triceps Kickback
Level 2, page 107

7. Wrist Curl
Level 1, page 112

8. Wrist Extension
Level 1, page 112

9. Advanced Bicycle
Level 3, page 81

everyday *secrets*

In the Game

Again ... warm up! You'll be running, jumping, twisting. You'll be rebounding, shooting, dribbling. If you don't stretch your muscles in advance and get your blood flow-ing, you greatly increase your risk of injury or serious joint and muscle pain afterward.

Keep it mellow. The NBA may be getting more and more physical each year, but we advise you to leave full-contact play to the pros. Smart defenders know that by keeping their hands high and staying between the players they are guarding and the hoop, they make it awfully hard for their opponents to get off a shot. No roughhousing is necessary. Be strategic, not aggressive.

Monitor your energy. If you find yourself standing around during the action, it is time to head to the

Instructions

Again, we propose a three-part workout—aerobic, strengthening, then stretching—three times a week. For the aerobic component, do 20 to 30 minutes of brisk walking, cycling, or light jogging, which mimics play on the court. Then do these 9 strengthening and 10 stretching moves. This part should take under 30 minutes. Start the strength exercises with one set of six repetitions. Try to hold your stretches for at least 15 seconds.

> Flexibility Exercises

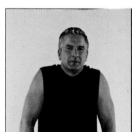 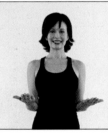 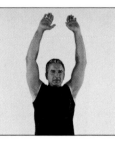 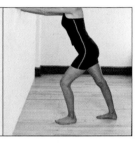 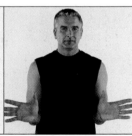

1. Seated Body Hang
Page 85

2. Lying Total Body Stretch
Page 77

3. Seated V
Page 53

4. Standing Quad Stretch
Page 54

5. Runner's Calf Stretch
Page 99

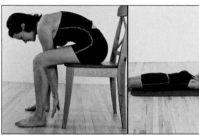 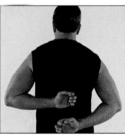 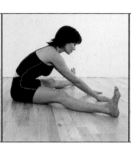 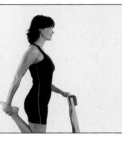

6. Shoulder Roll
Page 68

7. Knuckle Rub
Page 69

8. "Good Morning" Exercise
Page 70

9. Forearm Flip
Page 104

10. Handshake Wrist Bend
Page 110

bench for a rest. In a game, basketball players should be constantly on the go, getting clear for a pass or preparing to defend. Flat-footedness means you need a rest. Remember: Teams that win are the teams with energy, particularly come the fourth quarter.

Skip the game. There are many, many great basketball drills and games that are far easier on your joints than a formal game. Playing "21" from the foul line; having a game of Horse; even just lay-up drills or random shooting makes for a great time.

Make a clean shot. To improve your shooting, sometimes you just have to focus on setup and form, making sure your head and chest squarely face the basket, getting the ball into your favored hand just before release, and letting fly by flicking from the wrist, not pushing from the arms. ■

[11] Swimming

No matter what your age or health, swimming is a delight. It feels good, it's fun, and it's a wonderful way to exercise. Swimming mainly works your upper body. As a result, conditioning for swimming demands a lot of attention to range of motion and strength in the shoulders, back, and chest, with a still-important nod to exercises for the hips, legs, ankles, and feet.

> Strength Exercises

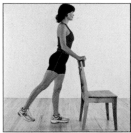

1. Standing Hip Extension

Level 2, page 60

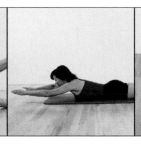

2. Side Thrust Kick

Level 3, page 63

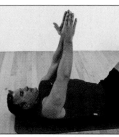

3. Superman

Level 2, page 87

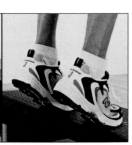

4. Chest Fly

Level 1, page 92

Stair Heel Raise **5.**

Level 2, page 100

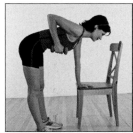

6. Bent Single Arm Row

Level 2, page 88

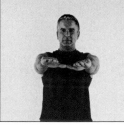

7. Around the World

Level 2, page 74

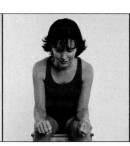

8. Wrist Rotation

Level 1, page 113

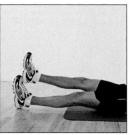

9. Flutter Kick

Level 2, page 79

everyday *secrets*

In the Pool

Position yourself. Getting through the water isn't merely a matter of generating power from your arms and legs. Instead, you'll slice surf easier (read: faster) by thinking of the shape your body makes as you move. Example: On a freestyle stroke, stretch your arm as far in front of you as possible after it enters the water (which the total body stretch will help you do) before pulling for power, to make your body longer and less resistant to the water.

Chafe at chopping. You're working hard, stirring up the water— but going nowhere. Don't mistake lots of effort for excellent exercise. You'll improve your efficiency and ultimately get a better cardiovascular workout if you focus on form, slicing your hand into the water on a freestyle stroke about

Instructions

Do these 9 strength exercises and 10 stretches two to three times per week to help prepare your body for swim time. As with the other routines, start the strength exercises with one set of six repetitions. Hold your stretches at least 15 seconds.

> Flexibility Exercises

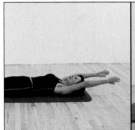 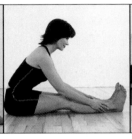 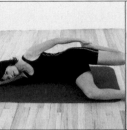 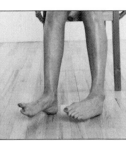

1. Lying Total Body Stretch
Page 77

2. Rocking Chair
Page 83

3. Straight-Leg Stretch
Page 53

4. Lying Quad and Hip Stretch
Page 54

5. Ankle Circle
Page 98

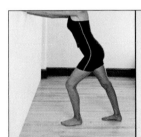 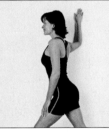 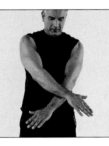 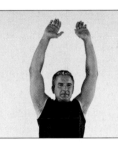 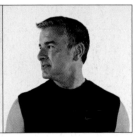

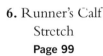

6. Runner's Calf Stretch
Page 99

7. Wall Side Stretch
Page 91

8. Scissors
Page 70

9. "Good Morning" Exercise
Page 70

10. Neck Turn
Page 94

eight inches short of a complete arm extension, and rotating your hips as you pull down and back.

Do a variety of strokes. To work muscles and joints from as many angles as possible, switch regularly from one stroke to another—such as freestyle, backstroke, breaststroke, and sidestroke.

Be playful. A swimming pool is a wonderful thing—great for your muscles, your joints, your heart, your spirit. So don't make your pool time all hard work. Walking through the water, treading water, bouncing on the bottom, diving for pennies, playing catch with a ball, just floating contentedly on your back—all are wonderful for your body. Even standing still and talking with a friend is better for your health when done in a pool. ■

Once you get the skiing bug, it never goes away. If weekend ski trips are the highlight of your winter, don't let arthritis slow you down. This program works the all-important hips, knees, and back, while also exercising upper-body muscles and joints needed to propel or support yourself with a pole. A bonus: By getting your body in shape for skiing, you make falls and wipeouts less damaging.

> Strength Exercises

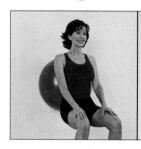 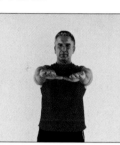 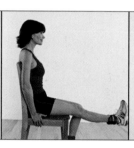 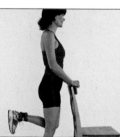 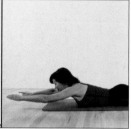

1. Ball Squat
Level 3, page 63

2. Around the World
Level 2, page 74

3. Seated Knee Extension
Level 2, page 62

4. Standing Knee Flexion
Level 2, page 60

5. Superman
Level 2, page 87

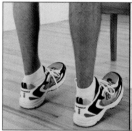 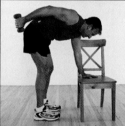 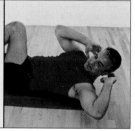 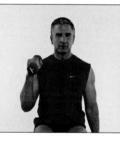

6. Heel/Toe Raise
Level 2, page 101

7. Triceps Kickback
Level 2, page 107

8. Hammer Curl
Level 2, page 107

9. Basic or Advanced Bicycle
Level 2 or 3 depending on variation, page 79 or 81

everyday *secrets*

On the Slopes

Stay loose. If you take a spill on the slopes, you'll come out better if you keep your body relaxed rather than fighting the fall, which makes muscles tense and more prone to injury. Try to get your feet downhill as quickly as possible, especially on a steep slope, so you're better able to brake and absorb the force of further falling.

Take it easy. If downhill skiing becomes too much of a challenge, switch to cross-country skiing. It may not have the excitement of alpine skiing, but it is easier on the joints and a better aerobic workout.

Focus on lateral movement. Skiing demands lots of side-to-side movements that aren't natural in everyday life. So if you are serious about preventing soreness and

Instructions

When ski season approaches, we recommend you do this three-part exercise program to get ready. Three times a week is best, for at least a month prior to hitting the slopes. First, do a cardiovascular workout: 15 to 20 minutes of cycling or brisk walking (both level and on hills, if possible), or climb stairs to build leg endurance. Then do the following 9 strengthening and 7 stretching moves. This part should take under 20 minutes. Start the strength exercises with one set of six repetitions. Hold your stretches at least 15 seconds.

> Flexibility Exercises

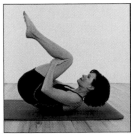 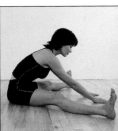 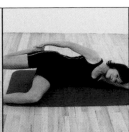 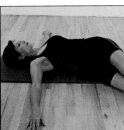 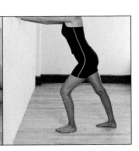

1. Rocking Chair
Page 83

2. Seated V
Page 53

3. Lying Quad and Hip Stretch
Page 54

4. Pelvic Twist
Page 83

5. Runner's Calf Stretch
Page 99

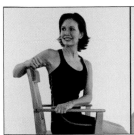 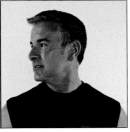

6. Seated Swivel
Page 99

7. Neck Turn
Page 94

avoiding injury, do sports or exercises that have you moving laterally. Even just a few minutes of shuffling sideways three or four times a week helps. Better is to line dance, play a little soccer with junior, or get in some tennis a few times a week leading up to ski season.

Work on your balance. Ultimately, skiing is about your ability to keep your weight upright and centered as your lower body moves through a wide range of motion. Balance starts in the torso, so be sure to exercise your abs and lower back well prior to ski season. In addition, do anything you can to practice your sense of balance—from standing on one foot to balancing on your toes. ■

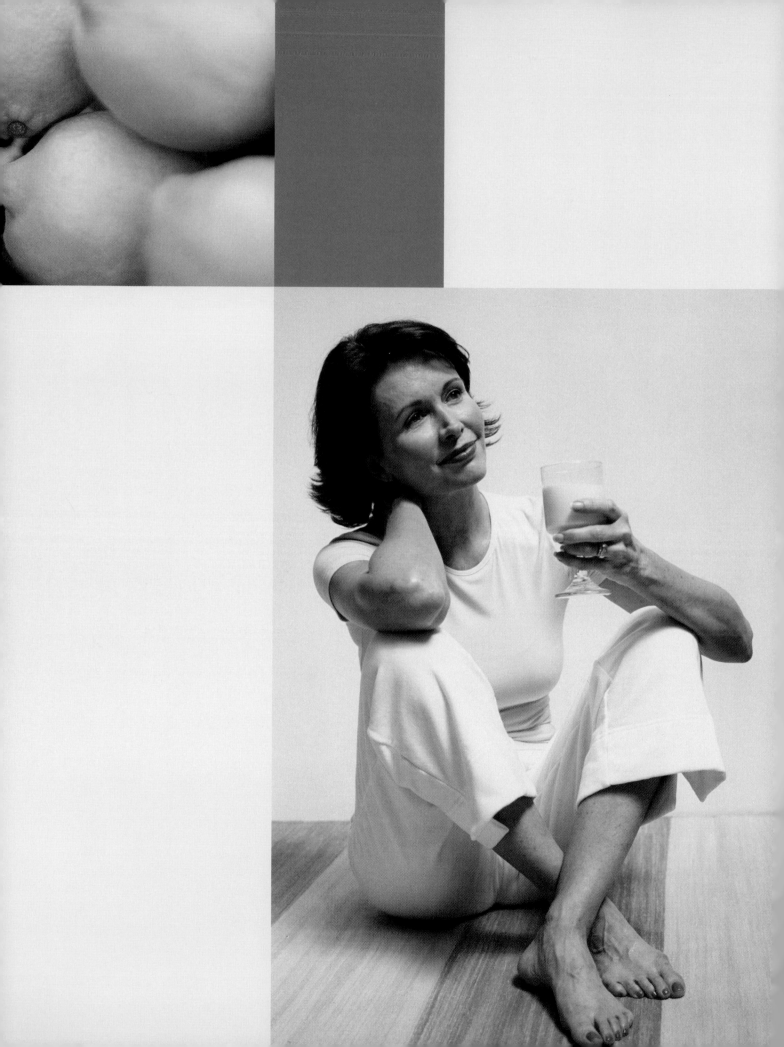

everyday food solutions

"You are what you eat!" is one of the oldest phrases in the lexicon of moms. Yet the message is as important for people with arthritis as it is for candy-gobbling children. In the pages ahead, you will discover foods and supplements that can indeed help you achieve healthier, less painful joints. You'll also learn the universal secrets of eating to lose weight, which is one of the best ways to alleviate arthritis pain. And best of all, you will encounter a dazzling assortment of simple and delicious recipes, each one rich with the nutrients you need to overcome arthritis.

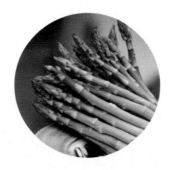

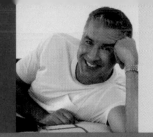
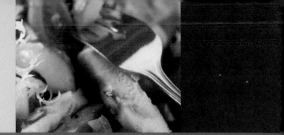

the best foods and supplements

I s there an arthritis diet? Your doctor would probably say no. The reason: Diet doesn't appear to affect arthritis to the same extent that it does heart disease, diabetes, certain cancers, and other challenging illnesses and conditions. As a result, no one has worked up exact guidelines, backed by decades of studies, on eating to beat arthritis.

Does that mean diet doesn't matter? Far from it. Even though there's much more to learn, compelling evidence suggests that eating a healthy diet—and even specific types of food—may help relieve arthritis symptoms or prevent arthritis from becoming worse. Lack of consensus may make precise diet prescriptions difficult, but making reasonable dietary choices at the very least can complement your exercise goals and improve your overall health. Here's how good nutritional choices affect arthritis:

- Getting more of nutrients believed to play a role in controlling inflammation may help ease symptoms, especially for rheumatoid arthritis.
- Making up for nutritional deficiencies sometimes caused by arthritis may help prevent joints from deteriorating further.
- Nutritional supplements such as glucosamine show promise in shoring up arthritic joints, although you should be cautious about self-medicating your disease.
- Losing weight by making smart food choices (along with burning calories with exercise) takes some of the load off joints, easing pain and slowing degeneration, especially with osteoarthritis.

There are no guarantees, and what works for you may not work for everyone with aching joints. But consider the possibilities: In one study from Denmark that controlled calories and boosted intake of arthritis-fighting foods, people who stuck out the diet showed significant improvements in morning pain and pain intensity overall, joint swelling, and medication costs.

SIX Key Anti-Arthritis Nutrients

The basic goal of good nutrition is to get enough of everything—which is easy if you eat a balanced diet that includes lots of different foods. But these six nutrients appear to have special benefits for people with arthritis. None of these nutrients offer miracle cures, and some appear to have more of an impact on arthritis than others. Bottom line: It's likely these nutrients help, getting more of them certainly won't hurt you, and it's easy to work them into your daily eating without overhauling your diet. Recipes starting on page 208 will show you how.

1. Omega-3 Fatty Acids

They may sound technical and unappetizing, but it's worth savoring what omega-3s do for the body— especially the joints.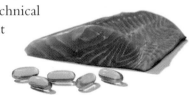
Fatty acids are a family of special fats that the body needs but can't make for itself, so you have to get them from food. Once in the body, they collect in cells, where they help form hormone-like substances, called leukotrienes, that put the brakes on inflammation— a root cause of rheumatoid and, to a lesser extent, osteoarthritis. More than a dozen reliable studies suggest that increasing your intake of omega-3 fatty acids can help quell symptoms of rheumatoid arthritis, even if the fats don't slow progression of the disease.

The most important food source of omega-3s is cold-water fish such as salmon, tuna, mackerel, and trout. But you'll also find types of omega-3s in nuts and seeds, beans, soy products, green leafy vegetables, and cooking oils such as canola oil. Fish oil is not entirely benign: Taking large amounts in supplements can have side effects, and even eating too much fish raises health concerns. Nor is cod liver oil the answer. It is high in calories, has high amounts of vitamin A, and may contain high amounts of cholesterol. Here's how to safely add omega-3s to your diet.

- **Switch from corn oil to canola oil.** Close relatives of the omega-3s are the omega-6s, fatty acids found in corn and other vegetable oils. While omega-3s (found in abundance in canola oil) are beneficial for your joints, omega-6s aren't: they make arthritis pain worse by promoting inflammation. They also compete with omega-3s in the body. So by switching your cooking oil, you boost your cells' usage of omega-3s and bring your body's fatty acids into better balance.

- **Consider omega-3 supplements.** To get omega-3s in the amounts used for many studies, you'd need to eat more fish than you can probably stomach—at least three servings every day. That makes taking fish oil supplements a viable alternative. But first, check with your doctor. On the whole, fish oil is safe, with mild side effects such as fishy burps. But omega-3 fatty acids also thin the blood, so you should be cautious if you're taking blood-thinning medications, including aspirin.

- **Emphasize salmon and canned tuna.** It's not that these fish are richer in omega-3s than their cold-water companions; it's that they are generally safer to eat. The Food and Drug Administration warns that many cold-water fish, such as king mackerel, swordfish, tilefish, and shark, contain toxic levels of mercury that make eating too much of them potentially dangerous. A safe limit: no more than 14 ounces a week of fish on the FDA caution list cited above. As for salmon, they are usually farmed or caught in the cleaner waters of Alaska. And cans of tuna tend to be packed with younger fish that haven't had as much time to accumulate toxins.

- **Say "no" if you have gout.** People with gout, a specific type of arthritis caused by excess uric acid, should avoid fish altogether because many types—including mackerel—contain purines, a building block for uric acid.

2. Vitamin C

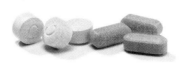

It's one of the most familiar of all nutrients, but vitamin C's role in joint health tends to be underappreciated. Vitamin C not only helps produce collagen, a major component of joints, but sweeps the body of destructive molecular byproducts known as free radicals, which are destructive to joints. Without vitamin C and other so-called antioxidant nutrients, free-radical damage to joints would be much worse. One of the best-known studies looking into vitamin C and arthritis, the Framingham osteoarthritis study, found that people whose diets routinely included high amounts of vitamin C had significantly less risk of their arthritis progressing. Points to bear in mind:

- **Drink OJ from frozen concentrate.** A prime source of vitamin C, orange juice is a favorite breakfast eye opener. While orange juice bought in the carton is wonderfully healthy, OJ made from frozen concentrate is even better. According to recent research published by the American Dietetic Association, juice reconstituted from frozen concentrate has more vitamin C than fresh-squeezed juice after four weeks of storage. If you prefer no-fuss pourable products, buy juice three to four weeks before the expiration date and drink it within a week of opening.

- **Spread out intake.** Your body doesn't store vitamin C; rather, it takes what it needs from the bloodstream at any given time and flushes out the rest. So a megadose in the morning doesn't really do as much good as you would think. Rather, replenish your vitamin C stores throughout the day by sipping citrus drinks or eating C-rich fruits and vegetables such as strawberries or melon, broccoli or sweet peppers at meals.

- **Beware of megadoses.** Your body needs about 60 milligrams of vitamin C each day for basic bodily functions. For healing and antioxidant purposes, many people take much higher doses. Most people aren't affected by a few hundred milligrams of vitamin C, but once you get past 500 milligrams or so, you should check with your doctor. Some people develop digestive unrest when they megadose on the vitamin. In addition, high doses of vitamin C can raise blood levels of salicylate medications such as aspirin, and can also interfere with absorption of other nutrients.

3. Vitamin D

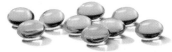

You can get vitamin D just from standing in the sun. That's because ultraviolet light converts precursors of the vitamin in the body into a usable form. Many people with arthritis are D-deficient. Studies find that getting more vitamin D protects joints from osteoarthritis damage, probably because this nutrient is vital to the health of bones that support and underlie joints. Vitamin D also appears to play a role in production of collagen in joints themselves. Some suggestions:

- **Get into the sunlight.** You don't need to bake on the beach to get sun-stimulated vitamin D: The skin only needs 10 to 15 minutes of exposure two to three times a week to synthesize what it needs. Your usual outdoor walks, games, or yard work should fill your vitamin D needs.
- **Read your dairy labels.** Milk, from skim to homogenized, is a prime source of vitamin D because it is D-*fortified*. Check labels on other dairy products. Though domestic cheese, cream, ice cream, butter, and yogurt often contain vitamin D, they're sometimes made with unfortified milk.
- **Beware of oversupplementing.** Vitamin D is a fat-soluble vitamin, which means excess amounts are stored in the body rather than immediately excreted. Large doses from high-potency supplements or multivitamins can build up and become toxic to soft tissues such as the kidneys and heart. Getting your D from foods and sunlight poses no such problems.

4. Vitamin E

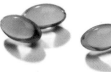

Like vitamin C, this is an antioxidant vitamin that protects the body—including the joints—from the ravages of free radicals. Some of the same research showing that other nutrients protect against arthritis also indicates that vitamin E can help prevent joints from becoming worse, though E's effects appear more limited than those of vitamins C and D. Some suggestions for getting vitamin E into your body:

- **Try soybean oil.** Up in the omega-3 section, we suggested switching to canola oil, which is widely available and no more expensive than corn oil. To go one better, though, try finding and then cooking with soybean oil. Though vitamin E can be tough to get from eating prime sources such as wheat germ and avocados, it's easy to pick up in other foods when cooked in this E-rich oil. Bonus: Soybean oil is also a good source of omega-3 fatty acids.
- **Combine with fish oil.** Taking vitamin E together with fish oil seems to boost the body's ability to fight inflammation beyond what either nutrient would do on its own, according to two recent studies in animals, at Loyola University, in Illinois, and the University of Buffalo. Be wary of heavy-duty supplements, however: Like fish oil, vitamin E thins the blood.
- **Compensate for cooking.** Whenever possible, eat E-rich foods raw—cabbage in coleslaw, for example. While a number of vegetables (including asparagus, brussels sprouts, and cabbage) contain small amounts of vitamin E, boiling can deplete food of as much as a third of its E content. Another option: Save cooking water, which retains leached nutrients, and use it to moisten mashed potatoes or make soup or sauce.
- **Add nuts to your cereal, salads, and snacks.** Sprinkling a quarter cup of almonds on your

breakfast cereal or lunchtime salad will give you your daily requirement of vitamin E. Pumpkin and sunflower seeds, eaten as a snack or added to muffins, are another good source of vitamin E. Of course, dieters should be careful. Nuts are as high in calories as they are rich in nutrients, so weigh the benefits and drawbacks.

5. B Vitamins

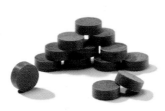

As cousin chemicals in the B-vitamin family of nutrients, vitamin B_6 and folate are also among the nutrients most likely to be lacking in people with arthritis. Part of this is due to deficiencies common population-wide—for example, one study found 90 percent of women don't get enough B_6 in their diet. But there's also evidence that the inflammation process eats up these B vitamins especially fast in people with rheumatoid arthritis—bad news for a variety of bodily functions, including the manufacturing of protein, the building block for tissues such as cartilage.

● **Double up.** When possible, eat foods that contain both vitamin B_6 and folate, such as spinach and fortified cereal. Otherwise, look to B vitamin sources for other arthritis-fighting nutrients. For example, in addition to being a rich source of B_6, tuna and sardines contain omega-3 fatty acids, and fortified cottage cheese contains vitamin D. Bonus foods for folate include asparagus (vitamin E) and broccoli (vitamin C).

● **Take a multivitamin.** To ensure you get enough of these nutrients, consider taking a multivitamin that provides 100 percent of the recommended Daily Value of 2 milligrams for B_6 and 0.4 milligrams for folate. (Look also for vitamin B_{12}, which works in tandem with folate.) But steer clear of high-dosage, single-nutrient supplements, which may pose risks of nerve damage.

6. Calcium

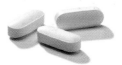

The issue with calcium, as with vitamin D, is bone health. Calcium has obvious importance to bones—more than 90 percent of the body's stores are contained in the skeleton and teeth. Getting too little calcium raises the risk of osteoporosis, a brittle-bone condition that accelerates if you have rheumatoid arthritis. All women (who are especially at risk) should get about 1,200 milligrams a day after age 50—about twice what's typical.

● **Drink milk; cook with milk.** You probably know that milk is a prime calcium source—but

HOW TO TAKE YOUR VITAMINS

Taking a multivitamin is the obvious approach to getting enough nutrients, but you'll benefit from putting some thought into supplements. Here are a few points for getting the most from your daily dose:

> **Take it with food**
The body is designed to absorb nutrients with real victuals, and it's easier to remember a multivitamin when it's a regular part of your mealtime ritual.

> **Choose reputable products**
Check for the stamp of the U.S. Pharmacopeia (USP), which sets voluntary standards for an otherwise unregulated industry.

> **Keep up to date**
The vitamins lining store shelves don't seem perishable, but they do lose potency. Check expiration dates and don't buy more than you can use in the time allotted.

> **Keep your balance**
If you're taking a multi, don't take other specific vitamins unless your doctor recommends it.

the same is true even for cooked foods made with milk. So consider having pancakes or waffles (one large waffle may contain as much as 12 percent of your daily calcium requirement) at breakfast or lunch. For other meals, balance your diet with low-fat cheese as a topping for savory fare such as chili or spaghetti.

- **Down it with D.** One reason vitamin D is so important to bone health is that it boosts the body's absorption of calcium—another reason to consume more D-fortified dairy, which contains both nutrients.

- **Go beyond the dairy case.** Milk and milk products aren't the only sources of calcium: It's also found in vegetables such as cauliflower, cabbage, brussels sprouts, kale, kohlrabi, broccoli, and turnip greens. These foods have less calcium than dairy products, but contain a form that's easier for the body to absorb. Other non-dairy calcium sources include omega-3-rich fish that have edible bones, such as salmon and sardines.

DO SOME FOODS MAKE ARTHRITIS WORSE?

Over the years, some arthritis sufferers have suspected that certain foods trigger symptoms or make them worse. Suspected triggers range from dairy, corn, or cereals to the nightshade family of plants, which includes tomatoes, potatoes, peppers, and eggplant. None of these ideas have been thoroughly studied, but

research suggests flare-ups people attribute to food are often actually due to some other cause.

So do your own test. If you suspect a food aggravates your arthritis, try eliminating the food for two to three weeks to see if you feel any better.

9 NINE Terrific Arthritis-Fighting Foods

It's easy to make arthritis-friendly nutrients part of a sensible daily diet because there's such a variety of them, covering virtually every food group. But with any nutrient, certain foods will always be richer sources than others. Below are super sources of the nutrients that battle arthritis best.

1. Salmon

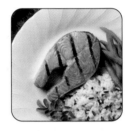

Salmon is among the richest sources of healthy fats, making it an ideal source of omega-3 fatty acids, especially because it's less likely than other cold-water fish to harbor high levels of toxic mercury. In addition to its fatty oils, salmon contains calcium, vitamin D, and folate. Besides helping with arthritis, eating salmon may protect the cardiovascular system by preventing blood clots, repairing artery damage, raising levels of good cholesterol, and lowering blood pressure.

- **Focus on freshness.** To avoid bacterial contamination, look for glossy fish that are wrapped to prevent contact with other fish. If you're buying fish whole, eyes should be clear and bright, not opaque or sunken, and flesh should not be slimy or slippery. Cuts like steaks and fillets should be dense and moist. In all cases, flesh should be firm and spring back if you press it.

- **Use quickly.** Fresh fish spoils fast, so if you can't eat salmon within a day after purchase, double its shelf life by cooking it right away and storing it in the refrigerator. (It is delicious served cold with cucumbers and dill.)

- **Tame total fat.** While you want the beneficial omega-3s in fish oil, the fat in fish is also loaded with calories. To keep from adding still more calories during preparation, cook salmon using low-fat methods such as baking, poaching, broiling, or steaming, and season with spices such as dill, parsley, cilantro, tarragon, or thyme.

- **Cook by color.** Following the rule of thumb for cooking fish—to wait until flesh is opaque white or light gray—is a tougher call with pink-hued salmon. To ensure doneness, cook salmon until it's opaque in its thickest part, with juices clear and watery, and flesh flaking easily with the gentle turn of a fork.

2. Bananas

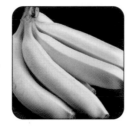

Bananas are perhaps best known for packing potassium, but they're also good sources of arthritis-fighting vitamin B_6, folate, and vitamin C. What's more, this easily digested, dense fruit is a prime source of soluble fiber, an important part of your diet if you're trying to lose weight because it helps you feel full without adding calories.

- **Control ripeness.** Bananas are sweetest and easiest to digest when brightly yellowed to full ripeness. To hasten or prolong the period of perfection:
  1. Put green bananas in a brown paper bag, which encourages natural gases from the bananas to speed the ripening process.
  2. Put rapidly ripening fruits in the refrigerator, which turns the peel brown, but preserves the fruit inside.

- **Preserve pieces.** Bananas are wonderful additions to salads or desserts, but tend to turn brown faster than other ingredients. Try tossing bananas with a mixture of lemon juice and water—the acid will help preserve them.

- **Turn into drinks.** Bananas, particularly ripe ones, make great blender drinks. Combine a banana, a peach or some berries, a few ounces of milk, a few ounces of fruit juice, and an ice cube, and blend for a delicious, healthy drink that is jam-packed with arthritis-friendly nutrients.

3. Sweet Peppers

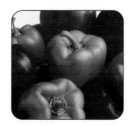

A single green pepper contains 176 percent of your daily needs for vitamin C—and colorful red and yellow varieties have more than double that amount. That makes them richer in C than citrus fruits, but sweet peppers are also excellent sources of vitamin B_6 and folate.

- **Lock in nutrients.** Store peppers in the refrigerator: The tough, waxy outer shell of bell peppers naturally protects nutrients from degrading due to exposure to oxygen, but you'll boost the holding power of chemicals in the skin by keeping them cold.

- **Separate seeds.** Whether cutting into crudités, tossing into salads, or stuffing whole, you'll want to remove tough and bitter-tasting seeds. They're easily cut when slicing, but when retaining an entire bell for stuffing, cut a circle around the stem at the top of the pepper, lift out the attached membranes, and scoop remaining seeds and membranes with a thick-handled spoon.

- **Jam them in the juicer.** You might not think of peppers as juicer giants, but they can add zest to drinks made from other fruits and vegetables, such as carrots.

- **Cook as a side dish.** Tired of the same old vegetables at dinner? Slice a pepper or two and do a fast sauté in olive oil, adding a pinch of salt, pepper, and your favorite herb. The heat releases the sweetness, making sautéed peppers a wonderful counterpart to meats and starches.

4. Shrimp

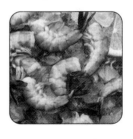

Taste and convenience make shrimp the most popular shellfish around. But shrimp also deserves acclaim as one of the few major dietary sources of vitamin D, with three ounces providing 30 percent of the recommended daily amount—more than a cup of fortified milk. Shrimp also contains omega-3 fatty acids and vitamin C, along with other nutrients essential for general health, including iron and vitamin B_{12}.

- **Select by senses.** When buying fresh raw shrimp, look for flesh that's moist, firm, and translucent, without spots or patches of blackness. Then put your nose to work: Shrimp should smell fresh and not give off an ammonia-like smell, which is a sign of deterioration. If you're buying shrimp frozen, squeeze the package and listen: The crunch of ice crystals means the shrimp was probably partially thawed, then refrozen—a sign you should find another (less crunchy) package.

- **Eat or freeze.** When you get shrimp home, rinse under cold water and store in the refrigerator for up to two days. If you plan to store beyond that, stick to frozen shrimp, which will keep in the freezer for up to six months.

- **Cook quickly.** Overcooking makes shrimp tough, so it's best to cook it fast, boiling in water until shells turn pink and flesh becomes opaque, stirring occasionally. Rinse under cold water and serve alone, as part of a seafood chowder, or chilled. Shrimp can also be broiled, grilled, or stir-fried.

5. Soy Products

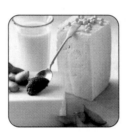

Once relegated to the shelves of health-food stores, soy products such as tofu and tempeh have reached the mainstream largely because they've been shown to have cardiovascular benefits. But soybeans also protect bones, thanks to compounds called isoflavones and significant amounts of both vitamin E and calcium. Long a staple of Asian diets, soy can also be found in soy milk—a boon for people who want to avoid lactose or cholesterol in regular milk.

- **Make the most of milk.** Use soy milk (now sold in many supermarkets next to cow's milk) for puddings, baked goods, cereal, shakes—just about anywhere you'd use regular milk. But don't mix it with coffee or other acidic foods, which tend to make soy milk curdle.

- **Try them whole.** Trust us: Whole soy beans, sprinkled with a little salt and pepper, are *delicious*. They look like large sweet peas but have an even gentler, milder flavor—nothing at all like the better known but more intimidating products like tofu. Check the freezer aisle for edamame (pronounced "ed-ah-MAH-may")—they come both in their pods, or shelled. They cook up fast—about five minutes in boiling water and two minutes in the microwave—and can be eaten hot or cold as snacks or appetizers, or tossed into salads, stir-fries, casseroles, or soups.

- **Give tofu a few more chances.** Many people don't know what to make of tofu. It's an odd color for a vegetable-derived food (white), an odd texture (smooth and moist), and comes in an odd form (usually, a block). Get past all that. Tofu is easy to work with, extraordinarily healthy, and takes on the flavors around it. Easy ideas: Drop half-inch cubes into most any soup; stir into tomato sauces, breaking it up into small pieces; or just cut into cubes, cover with chopped scallions and soy sauce, and eat at room temperature as is.

6. Sweet Potatoes

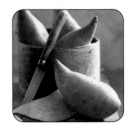

These tropical root vegetables (which, technically, not related to white baking potatoes) are such a nutritional powerhouse, they once topped a list of vegetables ranked according to nutritional value by the Center for Science in the Public Interest. Sweet potatoes are a rich source of vitamin C, folate, vitamin B_6, and dietary fiber, among other nutrients.

- **Buy fresh.** Though you'll benefit from eating sweet potatoes in any form, fresh potatoes are better than canned products, which are packed in a heavy syrup that leaches the vegetable's most valuable nutrients, including vitamins B and C.

- **Keep cool, not cold.** Store sweet potatoes someplace dark, dry, and cool—preferably between 55 and 60 degrees—but not in the refrigerator: Cold temperatures damage cells, causing the potato to harden and lose some of its nutritional value.

- **Maximize nutrients.** Eat cooked potatoes with their skin—an especially rich source of nutrients and fiber. Handle gently to avoid bruising, then bake or boil, and serve with a touch of fat from butter, oil, or another dish and some salt and pepper.

7. Cheese

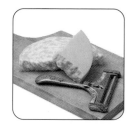

Hard or soft, fresh or ripened, cheese in all its variety is an excellent source of calcium for bones, and protein for muscles and other joint-supporting tissues. Depending on type, cheeses (especially hard varieties such as cheddar and Colby) are also a good source of vitamin B_6 and folate. The sheer abundance of cheeses makes it easy to get more in your diet—by, for example, slicing hard cheeses onto crackers or grating them into casseroles, or spreading soft cheeses such as cottage cheese or Brie onto fruits or vegetables.

- **Grease your grater.** When you have arthritis, grating cheese is hard enough without the grater becoming clogged. To make the job easier, give the grater a light coating of oil, which keeps the cheese from sticking and makes it easier to rinse the grater clean.

- **Lengthen shelf life.** Hard cheeses that are well wrapped and unsliced can last up to six weeks in the refrigerator. (Chilled soft cheeses are best used within a week.) To make cheese last even longer, throw it in the freezer, but expect thawed soft cheese to separate slightly and hard cheese to be crumbly—ideal for melting into casseroles and sauces but not as good for nibbling.

- **Let it warm.** Cheese tastes best when served at room temperature, so if you've been storing it in the refrigerator, take cheese out and let stand at least one hour before serving to enjoy its full flavor.

- **Have a daily cheese platter.** Healthy eaters know that every dinner table should have a plate of fresh raw vegetables in addition to all the prepared foods. Consider adding a large hunk of cheese to the platter each night, along with a knife. Sitting there in front of you, it's hard to resist slicing a piece off a few times to round out the meal.

8. Lentils

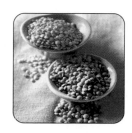

These dried legumes, with their rainbow of earthy colors, are prime sources of folate, with a single cup providing about 90 percent of your daily needs. But lentils also provide one of the richest plant-based sources of protein, contain large amounts of soluble dietary fiber, and hold significant stores of vitamin B_6. These and other nutrients make lentils protect the body against heart disease and cancer in addition to arthritis.

- **Try a few soups.** Not many people know a lot of lentil recipes. The most common usage—soup—is probably the best place to start for those new to the food. You might be surprised at how easy and tasty lentil soups can be. Add cooked lentils to water or broth, chop in carrots, celery, onions, and a lean meat, add some simple herbs and seasonings, and you are well on your way to a great meal.

- **Buy in bags.** Though sometimes sold in bulk from bins, it's best to buy lentils in plastic bags, preferably with most beans shielded from light. Reason: Exposure to light and air degrades nutrients (especially vitamin B_6) and open bins invite contamination by insects.

- **Pick the best beans.** Even bagged products aren't pristine: Sort through lentils before you use them by spreading them on a baking sheet and picking out those that are shriveled or off-color, along with any small stones that may have gotten mixed in. After that, there's no need to soak, but you should swish beans in a water-filled bowl, discard any floaters, and rinse under cold water in a strainer before cooking.

- **Minimize gas.** Thoroughly drain lentils before eating or adding to other dishes: Beans are famous for causing gas due to sugars they contain that the body can't digest, but these sugars are soluble in water and leach out when lentils are cooked.

9. Green Tea

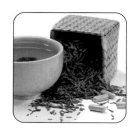

This mild, slightly astringent tea contains hundreds of powerful antioxidant chemicals called polyphenols and has been cited for helping prevent problems ranging from cancer to heart disease. But studies also suggest green tea may help prevent or ease symptoms of rheumatoid arthritis. In one study of induced arthritis in mice, green tea cut the disease onset rate almost in half, and follow-up studies by the same researchers, at Case Western Reserve University, in Ohio, show promise in humans.

- **Boil water briskly.** Tea tastes best when water is at the boiling point, which allows tea to release its flavorful compounds quickly. Water that's cooler than that tends to release flavors more slowly, weakening the tea.

- **Keep steeping short.** Let tea steep in hot water for about three minutes—and no longer than five. This brief steeping time allows tea to acquire a full-bodied flavor and release its nutrients, but withholds compounds that make tea taste bitter.

- **Get a bag bonus.** Tea purists favor the fresher flavor of loose tea, but some experts suggest that tea bags release more beneficial nutrients because smaller, ground-up particles expose more of the tea leaves' surface area to hot water.

TAKE THE TEA—DUMP THE DECAF

One study presented to a recent meeting of the American College of Rheumatology confirmed tea's arthritis-taming benefits: Older women who consumed three or more cups a day had a **60 percent lower risk of developing rheumatoid arthritis** than other women. But just as remarkable was a tandem finding that women who drank four or more cups of decaffeinated coffee a day appeared to double their risk of developing RA.

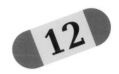

TWELVE Supplements to Be Aware Of

Anyone suffering from a chronic, painful condition such as arthritis is a prime target for sham treatments, and there's no shortage of over-the-counter remedies and herbs that claim they'll make your life "normal" again. But while it's smart to be skeptical, studies find that some remedies show promise for relieving pain and restoring mobility. Few supplements have been studied rigorously either for effectiveness or safety, however, and the fact that supplements are *not* FDA-regulated makes caution the byword. That's especially true when the market is lucrative: Americans spend more on natural remedies for arthritis than any other medical condition.

Keep in mind that quality and purity of supplements can vary tremendously, and always check with your doctor about side effects and drug interactions before starting to take any supplement regularly.

What follows here are details of 12 common arthritis remedies—products you will see at stores, discover through advertisements, or hear about through word of mouth. Unlike the nutrients we've just covered, we are not advocating you run out and get each of these. Rather, study the information, consult with your doctor, and make a clear decision about which you do or don't want to try.

1. Chondroitin Sulfate

Chondroitin sulfate—usually in combination with glucosamine—has been a popular arthritis remedy for years. But promising studies suggest that each of these supplements by itself may be effective at easing pain and improving joint function. Chondroitin is a natural component of human cartilage, but supplements are derived from cows or pigs. It's thought to ease symptoms of osteoarthritis by drawing fluid into joints to make them more supple, and by preventing enzymes from breaking down cartilage. More than a dozen studies, taken together, suggest it has benefits—results intriguing enough to prompt the National Institutes of Health (NIH) to launch a large study designed in part to reveal chondroitin's effects with glucosamine. Findings are due in 2005.

Chondroitin appears safe, but it may affect blood sugar and thin the blood, so approach it cautiously if you have diabetes or take anticoagulant medications. Don't expect instant results: Even people who say it works find that chondroitin can take as long as two to four months to have an effect. Typical dosing for chondroitin is 1,200 mg. a day divided into two or three equal amounts.

2. Collagen

Of two types of supplements that fall under this category, the most promising is collagen II, a natural component of cartilage. Usually made from animals such as chickens or cows, low-dose collagen II supplements are thought to relieve pain and stiffness from inflammation due to rheumatoid arthritis. One theory holds that introducing small amounts of supplemental collagen into the body causes attacking immune system cells to develop tolerance for your own collagen, making the immune system less likely to inflict more damage. Enough studies have suggested a positive effect from low doses that the National Institute of Arthritis and Musculoskeletal and Skin Diseases (NIAMS) has launched a two-year collagen II trial to be completed in 2004. Pending those results, collagen II generally appears safe unless you have an allergy to chicken or eggs. Dosage recommendations vary widely, but best results in studies so far have been from extremely small amounts: The NIAMS study is using between 30 and 130 mcg. a day. But supplements may not be necessary: You can also get collagen II from chicken soup.

Another type of collagen is collagen hydrolysate, sometimes known as gelatin, which is made by boiling the bones and skin of animals such as cows and pigs. Products containing gelatin have been promoted for arthritis based on the idea that amino acids in gelatin help repair and maintain joints. In one preliminary study, a powdered supplement containing gelatin, vitamin C, and calcium improved pain, stiffness, and mobility, but on the whole, claims for gelatin's benefits aren't well supported in the scientific literature. Still, though collagen hydrolysate may cause gastrointestinal trouble, it generally appears safe in typical doses of 10 grams.

3. CMO

This fatty substance, formally known as cetyl myristoleate, has been shown in an NIH study to prevent arthritis in mice (from which it's derived). Supplement makers have seized on this finding to bolster claims that CMO regulates the immune response responsible for conditions such as RA, fibromyalgia, and ankylosing spondylitis. But how it may work is largely a mystery, and there's no good evidence it is effective in humans. The Arthritis Foundation notes that research establishing safe dosage is lacking, and warns that some CMO promoters suggest you stop using doctor-prescribed arthritis medications to avoid blocking the effects of the supplement—a dangerous practice. For these reasons, many doctors recommend staying away from CMO.

4. Devil's Claw

The root of this herbaceous plant (named for the hooklike bumps on its fruit), is a traditional African pain reliever and a popular arthritis remedy, especially in Europe. Its active ingredient, harpagoside, is thought to be an anti-inflammatory agent—the basis for thinking devil's claw may help relieve pain and ease symptoms of arthritis, particularly RA. Much of the research on devil's claw has been done in Europe, where the German Federal Institute for Drugs and Medical Devices reports most studies to be poorly conducted and findings to be mixed. One of the best studies, however, found devil's claw to be effective against arthritis pain, though it's unclear whether the herb actually reduces inflammation or works in some other way.

Devil's claw, which comes in capsules, teas, and tinctures, appears to be safe even in doses above the 2 and 4 grams typically recommended. It's best taken between meals because stomach acids that peak after eating may hinder its effects. Caveats: Be careful if you have ulcers or diabetes, take blood thinners, or are pregnant: Devil's claw can stimulate the gastrointestinal tract and uterine wall, and may interfere with certain medications.

5. DHEA

Not a nutrient or herb, DHEA (dehydroepiandrosterone) is the body's most abundant androgen—a type of steroid hormone that's used to make other hormones, including testosterone and estrogen. People with rheumatoid arthritis have been found to have low levels of DHEA, prompting speculation that taking more in supplements might ease RA symptoms, especially since androgens are known to inhibit the body's immune response. Does DHEA work? So far, there's no direct evidence it actually controls rheumatoid arthritis, but a number of studies suggest it relieves joint pain and inflammation in women with lupus, another joint disease caused by immune system attack.

If you decide to try DHEA, ask your doctor to guide you—first of all, by finding a source of medical-grade products. Purity and dosage (which are always iffy with over-the-counter supplements) are particularly important with DHEA because it has potentially serious side effects. These may include raising risks of endometrial cancer and prostate cancer, and lowering amounts of "good" HDL cholesterol in blood. More immediate hormone-related side effects may include hair growth on the face and body, acne, deepening of the voice, and menstrual irregularities. Your doctor can also guide you on dosage: It's typical to take 200 mg. a day (the amount used in some lupus studies), but your doctor may want to start you on a lower dose.

6. GLA

Gamma-linolenic acid—an active ingredient in evening primrose oil, black currant oil, and borage oil—is a fatty acid that helps the body produce anti-inflammatory prostaglandins. Though it hasn't been thoroughly researched, several good, small studies find GLA can help ease joint pain or stiffness from rheumatoid arthritis by as much as a third. In one study, almost three-quarters of people with RA who took evening primrose oil were able to cut back on their NSAID medications. The Arthritis Foundation says that such findings make GLA worth a try.

GLA's long use as a remedy for RA (and other problems such as eczema and diabetic neuropathy) provides a long safety record in which there appear to be no serious side effects. The main drawback may be that, depending on the type of oil you take and the amount of GLA per capsule or tablet, you could need dozens of pills to reach recommended doses between 1.8 and 2.8 grams a day. Look for high-dose products, but check with your doctor before starting a regimen: Oils containing GLA can thin the blood.

7. Glucosamine

Like chondroitin, glucosamine is a natural component of your own joints, but supplements get it from animals—in this case, shellfish. Glucosamine also appears to be one of the most effective natural remedies for shoring up degenerating joints. One of the most recent well-controlled studies of glucosamine found that taking supplements for three years held back progression of osteoarthritis and relieved symptoms by as much as 25 percent. Numerous studies over the past two decades have found that glucosamine relieves arthritis pain as well as NSAIDs like ibuprofen—sometimes better—with fewer side effects. It's not entirely clear how glucosamine works, but it's thought to provide joints with extra proteins that actually build or maintain tissue. It may also act as an anti-inflammatory agent.

As with chondroitin, glucosamine can take as long as two months to produce results, but appears to be safe in typically recommended doses of 1,500 mg., which you can find in capsules, tablets, liquid, and powder that you mix into a drink. Though it's worth being wary of glucosamine if you're allergic to shellfish, it generally appears safe, with few side effects beyond mild gastrointestinal problems (which you may be able to remedy by switching to another brand). Check with your doctor, however, if you have high cholesterol, triglycerides, or blood sugar—glucosamine may raise levels of all three.

8. MSM/DMSO

MSM (methylsulfonylmethane) is a relatively recent arrival on the supplement scene, but DMSO (dimethyl sulfoxide), from which it's derived, has been touted as an arthritis remedy for decades. DMSO is an extremely versatile solvent that's used both for industrial purposes (it's in paint thinner and antifreeze) and medical applications (it's used to protect organs during transplantation, among other things). Though it is routinely used as an arthritis treatment in other countries, U.S. studies have failed to show any consistent benefit from medical-grade DMSO, and it's been out of favor since the 1960s, when animal studies found it may damage vision. Today, medical-grade DMSO is tough to find in the United States, and DMSO on the market is likely to be impure and potentially dangerous.

Enter MSM, which has been touted as the active ingredient in DMSO—only safer. Proponents say it's an anti-inflammatory that can ease symptoms of rheumatoid arthritis, and some studies have suggested a benefit in mice. But there's no scientific evidence that it works in people or that it's safe, even in the 1- to 3-gram doses typically used.

9. SAM-e

Popularly known as "Sammy," S-adenosylmethionine is a naturally occurring chemical with dozens of functions in the body. Often used as an antidepressant, it's also reputed to rebuild cartilage, hinder inflammation, and ease pain in people with osteoarthritis. It's long been available in Europe, where multiple studies have suggested SAM-e improves joint symptoms. In one large study, about 80 percent of arthritis sufferers taking SAM-e reported less pain. Other studies find it has pain-relieving effects comparable to many NSAIDs, though SAM-e works more slowly.

SAM-e generally appears safe in both human and animal studies. A typical full dose is 400 mg. three times a day, which may be reduced to 200 mg. when symptoms begin to improve. (Avoid high doses, which can cause gastrointestinal problems.) Though SAM-e isn't found in food, you may be able to boost your own natural production by eating green, leafy vegetables and other foods high in folate, which helps the body make SAM-e. Be sure to tell your doctor if

Other Armories of ARTHRITIS-FIGHTING NUTRIENTS

Omega-3 fatty acids
pecans
black beans
flaxseed

Vitamin C
broccoli
strawberries
tomatoes

Vitamin D
eggs
mushrooms
tuna

Vitamin E
spinach
asparagus
lobster

Vitamin B6
chicken
avocado
cantaloupe

Folate
corn
peas
kidney beans

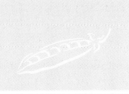

Calcium
sardines
turnip greens
black-eyed peas

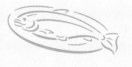

you start taking supplements, especially if you're on antidepressants, which may interact with SAM-e.

10. Shark Cartilage

If osteoarthritis makes you lose cartilage, why not replace it by eating more? That's one way to explain why taking supplements of cartilage ground from sharks or other animals might fight arthritis. But shark cartilage also contains collagen II, chondroitin sulfate, and calcium—all of which play a role in maintaining healthy joints or show promise in relieving arthritis symptoms. Preliminary animal and lab studies suggest that shark cartilage may indeed have anti-inflammatory and analgesic effects, but no well-controlled studies in people have yet shown it to have any impact on arthritis. Likewise, little is known about how much shark cartilage in capsules, tablets, or powder you should take, though per-pill doses on the market range from 250 mg. to 750 mg. The most common side effects include gastrointestinal problems such as nausea and vomiting, but shark cartilage has also been known to cause low blood pressure, dizziness, high blood sugar, and fatigue.

11. Stinging Nettle

Approved by the German medical establishment for treating prostate problems in men, supplements made from the stalklike stinging nettle plant are also said to reduce inflammation and ease pain from arthritis. In folk medicine, the irritating leaves of the plant were rubbed on the site of pain, which probably either triggered an anti-inflammatory reaction at the site or simply overrode one form of discomfort with another. Today fresh leaves have been replaced by extracts in capsules, teas, and tinctures designed to ease pain without irritation. Research suggests nettle supplements may work. One German study found that people who took a quarter dose of a prescription NSAID along with stinging nettle reduced pain from arthritis just as much as people who took the full drug dose. Other studies also find that taking stinging nettle can reduce your need for pain medication.

To use stinging nettle, take 1 to 4 ml. of tincture or make tea three times a day. To make tea, mix two teaspoonfuls (about 1.5 grams) of finely cut herb in water, boil, steep for 10 minutes, strain, and drink one cup.

12. Thunder God Vine

For thousands of years, extracts from roots of this Asian plant have been used in traditional Chinese medicine to reduce pain and inflammation that go with autoimmune diseases such as RA. Now science is catching up: A 2002 study funded by the NIAMS found that 80 percent of people with rheumatoid arthritis who took thunder god vine extract showed rapid improvement in their symptoms with minimal side effects. Lab and animal studies suggest the vine hinders production of chemicals that contribute to inflammation.

Though safe doses haven't been established by Western science, extracts of 30 mg. are typically used in research. If you try the extract, however, try to find a qualified practitioner of Chinese medicine for the right root-based preparation: Thunder god vine leaves and flowers are highly toxic.

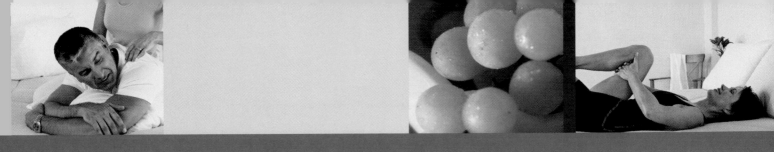

weight loss and arthritis

Losing weight: It's an American obsession. Bookstores, magazine racks, television talk shows, infomercials, billboards—you can't escape the latest diets, the outlandish promises, the ubiquitous before-and-after photos. It's hard to go through a day without encountering a weight-loss conversation. Many people are disgusted by it all. Why can't we just accept ourselves as we are? Who needs to look like a fashion model anyhow?

The disgust may be justified. The marketing of weight loss has gotten rather out of control, to the point that the federal government is starting to crack down on it all. But just because the marketing is excessive doesn't meant the goal of weight loss isn't desirable. It is, in just so many ways.

Weight loss isn't merely about vanity; it's about health. Particularly for people with arthritis, achieving a healthy weight can make all the difference in reducing pain and halting the advance of the disease. The primary reason is obvious: Carry around less weight, and you put far less stress and strain on your joints.

Being overweight with arthritis can become a vicious circle. Loading joints—especially knees—with extra pounds causes more pain and decreases mobility. That typically makes you cut back on physical activity, which in turn contributes to even more weight gain.

If you've started getting more physical activity to build strength and endurance, you've already taken a giant step toward breaking the cycle of increasing weight, pain, and disability. But most overweight people (and their doctors) recognize that exercise alone won't pare pounds. Instead, you need to combine your calorie-burning activity with diet control.

Losing weight can seem daunting, particularly with all the conflicting approaches and products being pushed at us. But the most effective diet tactics are deceptively simple. Better yet, they work best when you apply them over time rather than making a drastic overhaul of your current eating habits.

There's no doubt the changes are worth the effort. One of the most recent studies connecting weight and arthritis, a 2003 study of twins in Britain, found that about 56 percent of osteoarthritis is due to being overweight—a more significant role than genetics. But the fatness factor works in reverse as well, according to the Framingham osteoarthritis study, which found that dropping just two units on the body mass index scale (about 11 pounds for most people) cuts your risk of pain and stiffness by half.

Cutting Through the Controversies

Which diets take weight off best is the subject of heated scientific debate. No wonder: According to the Centers for Disease Control and Prevention, 64 percent of the U.S. population is now overweight or obese—a figure that has climbed steeply in the last decade and continues to rise. But it's important to recognize that, though there's much haggling over details (albeit important ones), there's also general agreement on a number of critical points.

For starters, weight-loss advice for decades has focused on cutting fatty foods mainly because doing so is an important way to cut risks of cardiovascular disease. As a result, "the public has come to think that eating too much fat is the only cause of overweight and obesity, which isn't true," says Robert Murray, M.D., who is associated with the Borden Center for Nutrition and Wellness at Ohio State University, and is a medical director at Ross Laboratories, a division of Abbott Laboratories. In fact, recent guidelines from the National Heart, Lung, and Blood Institute (NHLBI) state that reducing dietary fat alone "is not sufficient for weight loss." Instead, the consensus from NHLBI says the real issue is reducing calories. A key to doing it: Cutting back not just on fat but also on carbohydrates, which many people mistakenly believe are virtually harmless when it comes to weight loss.

Today the pendulum has swung all the way to the other side: Nearly every new weight-loss program focuses on a low-carbohydrate eating. The science of high-protein, low-carb diets like the Atkins program is complicated, having to do with the way your body processes nutrients, the nature of your metabolism, and the energy stores from which your cells draw their fuel.

But at the end of the day, no matter which diet you use, the basic problem is energy balance. To lose weight, you need to take in less energy (that is, calories) than you burn—by eating less, exercising more, or both. Even a small tip of the calorie balance can make a big difference over time. According to the NHLBI, the ideal diet leaves you with an average energy deficit of at least 500 calories a day (less than the amount in two peanut butter cookies), with a goal of dropping just one to two pounds a week. When weight loss plateaus, as it usually does after three or four months, exercise becomes especially important for maintaining losses and building muscle, which burns calories more efficiently than flab. Your weight loss may come slowly with these methods, "but if you're consistent, you'll make progress," says Murray.

How many of your calories should be fat versus carbohydrate? "What works best for you ultimately depends on what you can stick with and still reduce calories," says Murray. "Calories are where you make your stand." He recommends cutting back first on foods with heavy calories but little nutrition, such as cookies and ice cream—though you can indulge in them for the occasional treat or celebration. Next, get more vegetables (staples of both low-fat and low-carb diets) and whole-grain foods: They're rich in nutrients and fiber, which fills you up and keeps cravings at bay. Beyond that, Murray says, "there are a lot of ways to use food strategically."

WHAT'S YOUR CALORIE BUDGET?

Everybody's calorie needs are different, based on factors such as weight and activity levels. Your doctor or dietitian can help you figure exactly how many calories you should be eating every day, but there's also a way to come up with your own ballpark estimate. Here's how:

1.
Multiply your weight by 10. This provides a rough idea of how many calories your body needs when resting.

2.
Get an idea how many calories you typically burn with activity by using the following scale. If you're completely sedentary, give yourself 300. If you're moderately active, give yourself 500. And if you're very active, give yourself 700.

3.
Add the numbers from steps 1 and 2. This is approximately how many calories you need and can take in every day without putting on extra pounds.

6 THE SIX Key Tactics for Weight Loss

Some people need a rigorous, clearly defined program to keep them on the weight-loss path. Others just need to be pointed in the right direction. For those in the latter group, the following six tactics will give you the everyday secrets you need to start losing weight now.

Tactic 1: Cut Fat

Official recommendations still limit fat to 30 percent of your total calorie intake (with carbohydrate at 55 percent and protein at 15 percent) largely because fat contains twice the calories of the other nutrients. That means that cutting back on small amounts of fatty fare goes a longer way toward lightening your load than cutting the same amount of carbohydrate. But the kind of fat you eat is important as well. Saturated fat—the kind you're most likely to consume—is worst for overall health because it's most closely tied with cardiovascular risks.

Want an easy benchmark for knowing if a fat is saturated? Easy: if it is solid at room temperature, it's probably saturated fat. That includes butter, some cheeses, and the fat found on meats. These types of fat should account for no more than 10 percent of your total calories.

Other types of fat, such as arthritis-relieving omega-3 fatty acids and monounsaturated fats in oils such as canola, can actually be good for you. Bottom line, you should cut total fat mainly to avoid extra calories, and switch to healthier fats to improve your overall well-being and get more arthritis-fighting nutrients such as omega-3 fatty acids. Recommendations from the Arthritis Foundation include trading corn, safflower, and sunflower oils for olive, canola, and flaxseed oils, and eating no more than about two to four ounces of meat and poultry a day—an amount slightly larger than a deck of cards. Other suggestions:

- **Get milk.** Drink an extra glass of nonfat milk a day: It has two surprise benefits beyond bone-building. First, studies suggest that getting more calcium while cutting calories helps people lose more weight than they would by dieting alone. High calcium intake is linked with less body fat, lighter weight, and less weight gain in midlife. Second, getting more protein from milk or other sources can help you feel fuller on less food.

- **Take blubber from broth.** Skim fat from soups by throwing a few ice cubes into the pot: The fat will coagulate and cling to the ice after sitting a few minutes and come out of the broth when you take out the cubes.

- **Use your napkin.** Once heated, most fats are in liquid form. And that means they can be blotted off foods with a napkin or paper towel. So next time you get pizza, sop up the oil on top. With steak or meats, sop up the juices right before eating. When browning ground beef, pour out the oil and actually rub the meat down with a paper towel (being careful not to burn yourself!).

- **Cut the butter.** Butter is delicious, no doubt about it. But it is also almost pure saturated fat. Find ways to use less. Dip breads in olive oil or spread with fruit jam rather than buttering. Use salsa on baked potatoes. Experiment with low-fat or no-fat cream cheese spreads and herbs.

Tactic 2: Pare Portions

One reason Americans eat so many calories is that we tend to eat monstrous portions. Studies find that hamburgers and fries (to cite two notorious examples) are generally offered in serving sizes two to five times larger than the appropriate meal size. Not that we tend to care: Researchers find we usually clean our plates no matter how high they're piled, even if we already feel satisfied. Appalling-yet-appealing portions are one likely reason Americans continue getting fatter even as the percentage of our total calories from fat has gone down in recent years. Fortunately, portions are relatively simple to control because it's easier to count cookies than calories or grams of fat. To get a handle on the how-much factor, a first step is to eat out less: Restaurant portions are larger than most people serve at home, and you're more likely to eat fatty food when dining someplace special. But also check food labels when eating at home: Packages always list the calories in specific portion sizes—which may be smaller than you assume. Other suggestions:

- **Get pyramid particulars.** Go to the USDA website at www.usda.gov/cnpp/pyrabklt.pdf to download a booklet that explains serving sizes for the major components of the Food Guide Pyramid—which aren't spelled out on the pyramid itself.

- **Pre-picture portions.** Use familiar objects to picture how much you should eat of a food before you pick up your fork or spoon. For example, a half cup of low-fat granola is about the size of your fist. A half cup of low-fat vanilla ice cream equals half an orange, size-wise. And a serving of meat, chicken, or fish should be about the size of a deck of cards.

- **Consider the four-quarters rule.** Mentally split your dinner plate into four quarters. The perfect meal has a starch dish in one quarter, a protein in the second quarter, and vegetables in the remaining two quarters. Do that, and chances are you are close to the optimal mix of nutrients and food.

- **Use a smaller dish.** Sounds ridiculous, but it works. First and most obvious is that you can't put as much food on, say, a salad plate. But psychologically, you're just not as inclined to eat as heartily and quickly if your plate will be empty in 45 seconds.

- **Keep the seconds far away.** If you put the extra chicken or mashed potatoes on the table, all you have to do is reach over to get to them. If they are back in the kitchen (and even better, already put away) you'll be less inclined to gobble food mindlessly.

- **Have raw vegetables at every meal.** Raw cucumbers, tomatoes, carrots, peppers, and celery have few calories and lots of nutrients. A plate of them in the middle of the table almost always gets eaten up, cutting down appetite for the more calorie-dense meat or starch courses.

- **Start your meal with soup.** Studies show that a bowl of soup at the start of the meal reduces overall meal consumption. Consommés and brothy vegetable soups are best, since they are lowest in calories and highest in nutrients.

- **Manage your fork.** After every bite of food, put your fork down. Don't pick it up until you have thoroughly chewed and swallowed the previous bite. The goal is both to slow down your eating and to eat less. Remember: Your body needs 20 minutes of digestion before it sends signals to your brain that you are no longer hungry.

- **Have a snack.** Escape the trap of thinking you'll eat less if you quit noshing between meals entirely—the opposite is true. While you don't want to overeat, occasional snacking on low-calorie foods helps you feel satisfied and less prone to stuffing yourself when you finally sit down to a meal. Feeding small amounts of food into your system also keeps your energy up throughout the day and doesn't overload your digestive system at mealtime. Some ideal snacks: carrot or zucchini sticks with salsa, pretzels with low-sodium vegetable juice, and air-popped popcorn without butter. Get in the habit of two to three 100-calorie snacks per day.

Tactic 3: Sidestep Sugars

Avoiding sugar has always meant limiting sweets and soft drinks because they contain too many empty calories and too few nutrients. But now concerns about sugar have broadened to include other types of simple carbohydrates, especially quickly digested refined starches such as white bread and baked potatoes. Controversial eating plans such as the Atkins diet have long held that excess carbohydrates, not fat, are the true cause of weight gain. Once-skeptical nutrition researchers are beginning to take this possibility more seriously. In one recent study, published in *The New England Journal of Medicine,* people on a low-carb diet that included omega-3 fatty acids lost three times more weight than people on a low-fat diet over a period of six months.

The long-term effects of such diets aren't well studied, and it remains to be seen whether they're better at keeping weight off over time. "At this point, nobody can justify a dogmatic stance on where calories should come from," says Murray. But many researchers (notably a team at Harvard University's School of Public Health) endorse the idea of avoiding simple starches (including potatoes) and sugars, which may cause chemical changes in the body that lead to weight gain, in favor of whole grains, healthy fats, and lots of vegetables. Here are everyday ways to do so:

- **Rethink breakfast.** Pancakes, waffles, muffins, bagels, doughnuts—they're all big blasts of usually simple carbohydrates. Here's the perfect breakfast, for each and every day: one serving of fruit, one serving of dairy, and one serving of a complex carbohydrate. The dairy likely would be low-fat milk or yogurt. The carbohydrate, a slice of whole-wheat toast or a multigrain breakfast bar. Fruit is your choice.

- **Rethink dessert.** The old line is that you only get dessert if you clean your plate. Hmmm… sounds to us like a formula for obesity! Desserts are often filled with white flour, sugar, butter, and other tasty but empty calories. We suggest you clean your plate so you *don't* want dessert. Instead, consider dessert one of your two or three 100-calorie snacks for the day. Skip an immediate dessert, wait an hour or two after you finished dinner, and if you are truly hungry before bedtime, have the perfect dessert: a fistful of fresh strawberries. If not that, an orange.

- **Break the code.** When grocery shopping, check labels for terms such as fructose, maltose, lactose, sucrose, and dextrose—all of which indicate there's sugar in the food, even if the word "sugar" isn't highlighted on the front of the package. And don't be fooled by terms like "no added sugar," which can be used to disguise high amounts of natural sugar.

- **Forgo fructose.** Be especially on the alert for high-fructose corn syrup, a common sweetener that's loaded into non-diet soft drinks and many processed foods. It's not just the empty calories you're trying to avoid: Studies suggest high-fructose corn syrup fails to trigger hormones that regulate body weight and appetite.

- **Junk juices.** Replace fruit juice, flavored sports drinks, and soft drinks with plain or sparkling water, and add a wedge of lemon for flavor: By downing just one less sweet drink a day, you'll lower your calorie tally enough to keep off an extra 10 pounds in a year.

- **Gravitate to whole-grain.** Eat whole-grain foods that don't process out bran and fiber, such as whole-wheat bread—they contain more complex carbohydrates than foods made with refined flour, like white bread. Complex carbs are less rapidly absorbed by the body and are generally thought to pose less of a weight gain risk than the simple sugars more abundant in refined-flour foods.

- **Order it brown.** Many Asian restaurants now give you the option of brown rice or white rice. Choose brown rice: it is the whole-grain version that is much healthier and more filling than white.

Tactic 4: Tame Your Appetite

We tend to think appetite is the equivalent of the "empty" gauge on a dashboard: It lets you know you're low on fuel, so you stop to fill up. In practice, however, that's a better way of describing the mechanisms of hunger, which are different from those of appetite. Hunger is a biological drive to make sure you eat enough, while researchers say appetite has more to do with the choices we make based on learned desires. Appetite is a complex mix of body chemistry, habit, social behavior, and psychology that's notoriously difficult to manage. But the task isn't impossible, especially as researchers and therapists devote more attention to understanding the power of appetite and how to subdue it.

- **Ask yourself why.** For many people, meals aren't the reason we gain weight—it's all the nibbling and snacking we do in between. Experts point out that much of this kind of eating has nothing to do with hunger. Rather, it's boredom, or stress, or a learned habit independent of appetite (3:30 p.m.—time to get a snack at the vending machine!). There's a simple antidote: Ask yourself, honestly, why you are putting food in your mouth. If hunger is not the first reason, then stop.

- **Find alternatives.** So if so much eating is about boredom, stress, or habit, what to do when you are bored, stressed, or in need of a ritual? Easy: Take a walk. Put on music. Do a stretch routine. Go outside. Phone a friend. Read a favorite magazine. Knit. Yodel. Whatever gives you pleasure and relaxation. If you can create a new routine to deal with the everyday challenges that doesn't involve food, you will make major strides toward losing weight.

- **Turn on the lights**. When you wander into the kitchen at night, flip on all the lights. Research at the University of California, Irvine, suggests that you literally feel in the spotlight when you're brightly illuminated. The added self-consciousness and sense of being on display make you less likely to do things you shouldn't—like going on an ice cream bender.

- **Go to the candle store.** Next time you get a craving, light a scented candle: Studies suggest that certain aromas can take the edge off your appetite. The smells that work best include green apple, peppermint, and banana.

- **Pressure your appetite.** You won't find this in the National Library of Medicine, but when you feel weak-willed against your appetite, try pinching the small area of cartilage where your jaws hinge just below the ears, which some acupuncturists claim is an appetite control point. Hold for about half a minute.

- **Eat power pleasers.** To eat less at meals and snack time, choose foods that studies find have a high satiety index—meaning they're significantly more satisfying than other foods. Surprisingly, even though fatty foods fill you up and provide pleasure, they're not high scorers on the satiety scale because we tend to want more of them. Among the most satisfying foods: popcorn, jellybeans, potatoes, brown pasta, baked beans, grapes, and oranges.

Tactic 5: Make Small Lifestyle Adjustments

As we said earlier, lasting weight loss is more about small, sustainable adjustments to how you live and eat than it is following a rigorous, intense, short-term program that completely changes all aspects of your diet. The latter might deliver dramatic losses in the short term, but we all know how quickly the pounds can return once we get back into our everyday habits. We've already given lots of tricks and secrets to tweak how you snack, cook, and eat. Here are a handful more that can give your weight-loss efforts the edge you need to succeed:

- **Forget weight.** Too many people focus on pounds when it comes to measuring weight loss. Instead, focus on better measures: how your energy levels are doing, how your joints are feeling, how your attitude is faring, how your clothes are fitting, how you look in the mirror. Sure, your weight is the clearest measurement of your progress, but your goal shouldn't be a number: It should be measured by your health and happiness. If your joints are telling you your weight-loss efforts are helping, then there's no better measurement you could have.

- **Develop movement habits.** Research shows that people who fidget burn 500 or more extra calories in a day. Learn the lesson: all extra movements burn calories. So develop movement habits. Some examples: Stand when on the phone; leave the room during TV commercials; walk 10 minutes after dinner; tap your foot to the music. Develop one or two such habits, and you'll burn many more calories.

- **Drink water**. You've heard the health benefits of water just so many times. So finally do it: Get yourself a big, interesting, friendly cup or Mason jar or travel mug, fill it up after breakfast, and keep it with you everywhere. Refill, refill, refill. At the end of the day, wash it out and have it ready for tomorrow. Nothing will satiate your hunger as well as plentiful cool water.

- **Entertain your mouth.** Sometimes all it takes to halt the snacking is a piece of gum, a slow-to-dissolve piece of candy, a toothpick, even an olive pit. While society looks down on overt mouth habits in public, if you can be subtle, there's absolutely nothing wrong with an hour-long engagement with a piece of sugarless gum, particularly if it keeps you from snacking.
- **Shop the perimeter.** Big grocery stores are laid out in predictable ways. Usually, the healthiest, freshest foods are around the perimeter: produce, meats, seafood, dairy, bakery. The danger is in the aisles, with its cookies, potato chips, canned foods, boxed foods, ice creams, and such. Your food-shopping goal: Stay only along the store perimeter. Just once a month, delve into the aisles for necessary staples.
- **Spice up your meals.** Add zest to food with cayenne and jalapeño peppers, ginger, Tabasco sauce, mustard, and other spices. Studies find that zingier foods have thermogenic properties that boost your metabolism's fat-burning ability—by as much as 25 percent, in some reports.
- **Sleep better.** It sounds like quackery, but you really can encourage weight loss by sleeping. Research into sleep and hormone function finds that your metabolism rises and you burn calories more efficiently when you're well rested.
- **Nix Nickelodeon.** Avoid the TV programs you enjoy with your kids or grandkids—or tune out the commercials. Children's programming contains much more junk food advertising than adult shows: 2,800 calories per hour, on average, according to researchers at the University of California, Davis. And studies find that watching less food on the tube translates to fewer fatty, sweet products in pantries.
- **Top your tank before exercise.** Have a well-balanced carbohydrate/protein snack such as half an apple with peanut butter or crackers with low-fat cheese an hour or more before a workout. The carbs will keep energy high while you exercise, and the protein will slow your digestion, giving you stamina for sustained effort.
- **Skip the wine.** If you sip a glass of wine or beer with meals, think about a prohibition diet. The drink isn't bad per se, but your body tends to give priority to processing alcohol, making calories from the food you eat more likely to be stored as fat, according to researchers at Pennsylvania State University.
- **Do the ring test.** Should you cut back your portions of salt? Even if you don't have high blood pressure, try this test: Slip a ring on your finger. Now eat salty food, wait a few hours, and try to take the ring off. If sliding the ring is more difficult now than earlier, you're probably among the many people (mainly women) for whom salt causes bloat—potentially grounds for several extra pounds, according to researchers at the University of Maryland. Check food labels for sodium and cut your intake to feel lighter on your feet.

Tactic 6: Eat Well—and Enjoy Eating!

When it comes to managing arthritis, fixing a good meal is no different from choosing the right medicine, enjoying healthy exercise, and keeping a positive attitude. All are integral to the everyday arthritis solution.

Developing a love of food that not only tastes good but is good for you can take practice and a guiding hand. The recipes that follow in the "Recipes for Beating Arthritis" section have been chosen because they are all rich in the nutrients that are so important to joint health, particularly the vitamins, minerals, and omega-3 fatty acids we've discussed. Better yet, they are all modest in calories, meaning they are perfect for people seeking to lose weight. Best of all, they are flavorful, creative, easy to prepare, and oh-so-yummy. While cooking these recipes won't give you instantaneous arthritis relief, they will give you immediate pleasure. Over time, a consistent diet of this type of eating can lead to significant joint improvement.

RECIPES FOR BEATING ARTHRITIS

Asparagus & Red Pepper Frittata

Asparagus and olive oil add vitamin E to this lovely brunch dish; the red bell pepper adds vitamin C, and the cheese supplies calcium. All make this a powerhouse anti-arthritis recipe.

PREPARATION TIME: 10 MINUTES
COOKING TIME: 20 MINUTES • **SERVES 4**

1/2	pound asparagus, trimmed and cut into 1/2-inch lengths
1	red bell pepper, cut into 1/2-inch squares
3	eggs
4	egg whites
2	teaspoons flour
1/2	cup grated Parmesan cheese
1/2	teaspoon salt
1/4	teaspoon black pepper
2	teaspoons olive oil
1	teaspoon unsalted butter

1. In medium pot of boiling water, cook asparagus and bell pepper for 2 minutes to blanch; drain well.

2. In medium bowl, whisk together whole eggs and egg whites. Whisk in flour until well combined. Whisk in Parmesan cheese, salt, and black pepper. Stir in asparagus and bell pepper.

3. In 10-inch cast-iron or other broilerproof skillet, heat oil and butter over low heat until butter has melted. Pour in egg mixture and cook without stirring for 15 minutes or until eggs are set around the edges and almost set in center. Meanwhile, preheat broiler.

4. Broil frittata 6 inches from heat for 1 to 2 minutes or until top is just set. Cut into wedges and serve hot, warm, or at room temperature.

Calories: 170, fat: 10 g, saturated fat: 4 g, sodium: 530 mg, carbohydrate: 6 g, protein: 15 g.

Blueberry & Cranberry Granola

This delicious toasted cereal is made from a mix of vitamin E-rich grains, nuts, and seeds, and vitamin C-rich berries. Canola oil adds omega-3 fatty acids. Stirring maple syrup and orange juice into the granola helps to keep the oil content down, making this version much lower in calories than most "crunchy" cereals you buy.

PREPARATION TIME: 40–50 MINUTES, PLUS COOLING • **MAKES ABOUT 8 SERVINGS**

2 3/4	cups oatmeal
1/2	cup wheat germ
7	tablespoons millet flakes
2	tablespoons sunflower seeds
2	tablespoons slivered almonds
1	tablespoon sesame seeds
1/2	cup dried blueberries
1/2	cup dried cranberries
1	tablespoon soft light brown sugar
2	tablespoons maple syrup
2	tablespoons canola oil
2	tablespoons orange juice

1. Preheat oven to 325°F. In large bowl, combine oats, wheat germ, millet flakes, sunflower seeds, almonds, sesame seeds, dried berries, and sugar. Stir until well mixed.

2. In measuring cup, whisk together maple syrup, oil, and orange juice. Pour mixture slowly into dry ingredients, stirring until liquid is evenly distributed and coats everything lightly.

3. In a nonstick roasting pan, spread out mixture evenly. Bake until slightly crisp and lightly brown, 30 to 40 minutes, stirring every 10 minutes to encourage even browning.

4. Remove roasting pan from oven and leave granola to cool. Store in airtight container up to 2 weeks. Serve with plain yogurt, milk, or fruit juice.

Calories: 250, fat: 7 g, saturated fat: 1 g, sodium: 5 mg, carbohydrate: 45 g, protein: 6 g.

Whole-Wheat Breakfast Muffins

Muffins are always welcome at breakfast; these have low-fat yogurt for calcium, wheat germ for vitamin E, canola oil for omega-3 fatty acids, and orange juice and zest for vitamin C.

PREPARATION TIME: 15 MINUTES **COOKING TIME:** 15–20 MINUTES • **MAKES 12 MUFFINS**

2/3	cup whole-wheat flour
3/4	cup plus 2 tablespoons all-purpose flour
2	teaspoons baking soda
	Pinch salt
1/4	teaspoon cinnamon
1/4	cup packed dark brown sugar
5	tablespoons wheat germ
1	cup packed raisins
1	cup plain low-fat yogurt
4	tablespoons canola oil
1	large egg
	Grated zest of 1/2 orange
3	tablespoons orange juice

1. Preheat oven to 400°F. Grease 12-cup muffin pan.

2. Sift whole-wheat and all-purpose flours, baking soda, salt, and cinnamon into large bowl, tipping in any bran left in the sieve. Stir in sugar, wheat germ, and raisins, and make a well in the middle.

3. In small bowl, lightly whisk together yogurt, oil, egg, orange zest, and juice. Pour liquid ingredients into well in flour mixture and stir together just enough to moisten dry ingredients. Don't beat or overmix.

4. Spoon batter into muffin pan, filling each cup 2/3 full. Bake until muffins are just firm to the touch, 15 to 20 minutes. Leave muffins to cool in tray 2 to 3 minutes, then turn out onto wire rack. The muffins are best still warm from the oven. Leftover muffins can be cooled completely and stored in an airtight container up to 2 days.

Calories: 190, fat: 6 g, saturated fat: 1 g, sodium: 240 mg, carbohydrate: 20 g, protein: 5 g.

Eggs in Tortilla Flowers

Vitamin D from the eggs, vitamin C from the red pepper, and omega-3s from the canola oil make this a powerful starter for the day.

PREPARATION TIME: 15 MINUTES
COOKING TIME: 20 MINUTES • **SERVES 4**

	Nonstick cooking spray
4	corn tortillas, 6 inches in diameter
2	teaspoons canola oil
6	large eggs
4	large egg whites
2	tablespoons water
1/4	teaspoon black pepper, or to taste
1	large sweet red pepper, cored, seeded, and finely chopped (1 cup)
4	ounces reduced-sodium ham, finely cubed (1/2 cup)
2	scallions, including tops, sliced
	Salsa (optional topping)

1. Preheat oven to 325°F. On baking sheet, invert 4 small custard cups or ovenproof glasses and coat bottoms with nonstick cooking spray. Brush each tortilla with 1/4 teaspoon oil, then cut 8 evenly spaced 2-inch-deep slits around the edge. Center each tortilla, oiled side up, on top of a cup, letting cut edges drape down sides. Bake for 20 minutes or until crisp.

2. After tortillas have baked for 10 minutes, start eggs. In medium bowl, beat together eggs, egg whites, water, and black pepper. In 10-inch non-stick skillet over moderately low heat, heat remaining oil. Add red pepper, ham, and scallions. Cover and cook for 6 minutes or until softened.

3. Add egg mixture and cook, uncovered, 3 minutes more, scrambling eggs lightly until they are just set. Remove tortillas from the custard cups and invert them on 4 individual serving plates. They will have formed shallow, flowerlike cups. Fill each tortilla flower with egg mixture and serve immediately. Top with salsa if desired.

Calories: 270, fat: 13 g, saturated fat: 3 g, sodium: 460 mg, carbohydrate: 19 g, protein: 20 g.

Orange-Banana Breakfast Smoothie

Vitamin C from the orange juice and vitamin B$_6$ from the banana make this a most refreshing eye opener.

PREPARATION TIME: 5 MINUTES • **SERVES 1**

- 3/4 cup orange juice
- 1/2 cup sliced banana
- 2 teaspoons brown sugar
- 1/8 teaspoon almond extract.
- 2 ice cubes
  Mint sprig

1. In blender, combine orange juice, banana, sugar, and almond extract.

2. Add ice cubes and blend until thick and smooth.

3. Garnish with mint sprig.

Calories: 190, fat: 0 g, saturated fat: 0 g, sodium: 0 mg, carbohydrate: 46 g, protein: 2 g.

Strawberry-Yogurt Smoothie

This refreshing drink provides a healthy start to the day, with its high vitamin C and calcium content and natural sweetness. Dilute it with extra orange juice if you want a thinner drink.

PREPARATION TIME: 5 MINUTES • **SERVES 4**

- 1 pound ripe strawberries, hulled
  Grated zest and juice of 1 large orange
- 2/3 cup plain low-fat yogurt
- 1 tablespoon sugar, or to taste (optional)
- 4 small strawberries (optional)
- 4 small orange slices (optional)

1. Put strawberries into food processor or blender. Add zest, juice, and yogurt. Puree, scraping down sides of container once or twice. Taste mixture and sweeten with sugar, if necessary.

2. Pour into glasses. If you like, decorate with small strawberries and slices of orange, both split so they sit on the rim of the glass.

Calories: 90, fat: 0 g, saturated fat: 0 g, sodium: 35 mg, carbohydrate: 17 g, protein: 3 g.

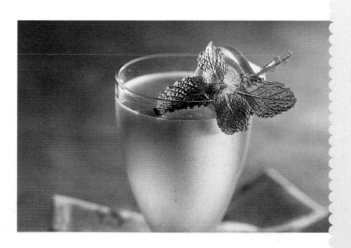

Black Bean Soup

Black beans are high in folate and calcium; bell peppers and tomatoes are high in vitamin C. This soup is, therefore, as healthy as it is delicious.

PREPARATION TIME: 5 MINUTES
COOKING TIME: 7 MINUTES • **SERVES 4**

- 1 diced green bell pepper
- 2 sliced scallions
- 3 cloves minced garlic
- 2 teaspoons oil
- 1 can (19 ounces) black beans, rinsed and drained
- 1 1/2 cups chicken broth
- 1 teaspoon each ground coriander and cumin
- 2 tablespoons reduced-fat sour cream
- 1/4 cup diced tomato.

1. In saucepan, sauté bell pepper, scallions, and garlic in oil until soft.

2. Add black beans, chicken broth, coriander, and cumin. Simmer 5 minutes.

3. In blender or food processor, puree half the soup and return to pan; reheat soup. Top with sour cream and tomato.

Calories: 180, fat: 5 g, saturated fat: 1 g, sodium: 460 mg, carbohydrate: 24 g, protein: 10 g.

Chunky Beet, Potato, & Beef Soup

Here's a healthy, hearty version of borscht, the famous Eastern European beet soup. The beets are full of folate and vitamin C, and the potatoes contribute vitamins C and B_6.

PREPARATION TIME: 30 MINUTES
COOKING TIME: 35 MINUTES • **SERVES 4**

- 2 teaspoons olive oil
- 6 scallions, thinly sliced
- 4 cloves garlic, minced
- 2 1/2 pounds fresh beets, peeled and cut into 1/2-inch cubes
- 3/4 pound all-purpose potatoes, peeled and cut into 1/2-inch cubes
- 2 carrots, thinly sliced
- 1/4 cup red wine vinegar
- 4 teaspoons sugar
- 1 teaspoon salt
- 1/4 teaspoon pepper
- 3/4 pound well-trimmed top round beef steak, cut into 1/4-inch chunks
- 1/4 cup reduced-fat sour cream

1. In large saucepan, heat oil over moderate heat. Add scallions and garlic, and sauté for 2 minutes or until the scallions are tender.

2. Add beets, potatoes, carrots, vinegar, sugar, salt, pepper, and 4 1/2 cups of water. Bring to a boil, reduce to a simmer, cover, and cook for 15 minutes or until beets and potatoes are almost tender. Add beef and cook for 15 minutes or until just cooked through. Serve topped with a dollop of sour cream.

Calories: 440, fat: 8 g, saturated fat: 5 g, sodium: 760 mg, carbohydrate: 55 g, protein: 38 g.

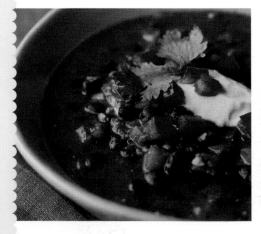

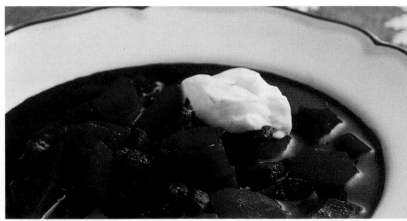

Creamy Cabbage & Carrot Soup

You can make this soup with crinkly Savoy cabbage, which is rich in folate and vitamin C. The carrots and tomato paste add more vitamin C. The sour cream contributes calcium.

PREPARATION TIME: 15 MINUTES
COOKING TIME: 40 MINUTES • **SERVES 4**

1	tablespoon olive oil
1	large onion, finely chopped
4	cloves garlic, minced
2	carrots, thinly sliced
8	cups shredded green cabbage
2 1/2	cups chicken broth
3/4	cup snipped fresh dill
1/3	cup no-salt-added tomato paste
3/4	teaspoon ground ginger
1/4	teaspoon each salt and pepper
1/3	cup reduced-fat sour cream

1. In large Dutch oven or flameproof casserole, heat oil over moderate heat. Add onion and garlic, and sauté for 7 minutes or until the onion is soft. Add carrots and sauté for 5 minutes or until the carrots are crisp-tender.

2. Stir in cabbage, cover, and cook, stirring occasionally, for 10 minutes or until cabbage is wilted.

3. Add broth, 2 1/2 cups of water, dill, tomato paste, ginger, salt, and pepper. Bring to a boil, reduce to a simmer, cover, and cook for 15 minutes or until cabbage is very tender. Stir sour cream into soup.

Calories: 180, fat: 9 g, saturated fat: 3 g, sodium: 810 mg, carbohydrate: 22 g, protein: 5 g.

Lemony Lentil Soup

This sturdy, healthy winter soup has a delicious citrus overtone combined with the warm flavors of roasted spices. The lentils provide you with almost a day's requirement of folate as well as some vitamin B_6. The lemon juice gives you vitamin C.

PREPARATION TIME: 5 MINUTES
COOKING TIME: 35 MINUTES • **SERVES 4**

1	tablespoon olive oil
3	cloves garlic, chopped coarse
1	medium onion, chopped
1 1/3	cups red lentils, rinsed and drained
4	cups chicken or vegetable broth
1	teaspoon ground coriander
1/2	teaspoon ground cumin
	Juice of 1 lemon
4	wafer-thin slices of lemon

1. In large heavy saucepan over medium heat, cook garlic and onions in oil until brown, 3 to 5 minutes. Add lentils and cook, stirring, for 2 minutes. Stir in broth. Simmer soup, covered, until lentils are almost soft, 15 to 20 minutes.

2. In dry skillet set over high heat, toast coriander and cumin until aromatic, 1 to 2 minutes, then add to soup. Add lemon juice, lemon slices, and salt and pepper to taste, and simmer soup for 5 minutes before serving.

Calories: 280, fat: 5 g, saturated fat: 1 g, sodium: 130 mg, carbohydrate: 41 g, protein: 18 g.

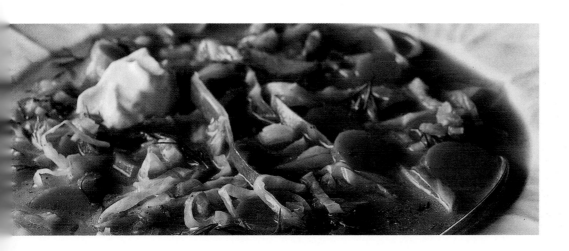

Portuguese Kale Soup

Rich in calcium and vitamin C, kale tastes great teamed with sausage, potatoes (with their vitamin C and B6), and kidney beans (good sources of folate and vitamin B6).

PREPARATION TIME: 20 MINUTES **COOKING TIME:** 45 MINUTES • **MAKES SIX 1 1/2-CUP SERVINGS**

4	ounces spicy turkey sausage or Italian sausage
1 1/2	ounces sliced pepperoni, slivered
1	large yellow onion, quartered and thinly sliced (1 1/2 cups)
1	medium stalk celery, coarsely chopped (1/2 cup)
1	can (14 1/4 ounces) low-sodium chicken broth mixed with 6 cups water
8	ounces kale, thick stems removed and leaves sliced (about 8 cups), or 2 packages (10 ounces each) frozen kale, thawed and squeezed dry
1/2	teaspoon minced garlic
12	ounces red-skin potatoes, halved and sliced (2 cups)
1/2	teaspoon hot red pepper sauce, or to taste
1/4	teaspoon salt, or to taste
1 1/2	cups cooked red kidney beans

1. Remove casings from sausage and discard; crumble the meat. In stockpot or 5-quart Dutch oven over moderately low heat, cook sausage, stirring, for 4 minutes. Add pepperoni and cook 2 minutes more or until fat is rendered. Drain sausage and pepperoni on paper towels. Pour out all but 1 teaspoon of fat from stockpot and discard.

2. Add onion and celery to stockpot and cook over low heat, covered, stirring occasionally, for 8 minutes or until softened. Return sausage to stockpot and add stock, kale, and garlic. Bring to a simmer, cover, and cook for 10 minutes.

3. Stir in potatoes, red pepper sauce, and salt. Simmer, covered, 20 minutes more or until potatoes and kale are tender. Add beans and cook just until heated through.

Calories: 229, fat: 7 g, saturated fat: 2 g, sodium: 498 mg, carbohydrate: 30 g, protein: 13 g.

Sweet Corn Chowder

Corn is high in folate, the seasoning vegetables add vitamin C, and the milk adds calcium to this all-time favorite soup that is actually good for you!

PREPARATION TIME: 20 MINUTES
COOKING TIME: 45 MINUTES • **MAKES 11 CUPS**

2	ounces reduced-sodium bacon, coarsely chopped
2	large onions, diced
2	large carrots, diced
2	stalks celery, diced
12	ounces all-purpose potatoes, peeled and diced
6	cups chicken stock
2	cups fresh or frozen corn kernels
2	cups 1% low-fat milk
1/8	teaspoon each salt and pepper
	Cayenne pepper

1. In 4-quart saucepan over moderate heat, cook bacon until browned and fat rendered, about 4 minutes. Remove bacon with slotted spoon and reserve for garnish.

2. Add onions, carrots, and celery to saucepan and sauté until softened, about 5 minutes..

3. Stir in potatoes with chicken stock and bring to boil. Simmer soup, partially covered, stirring occasionally, until the vegetables are tender, about 10 minutes.

4. Add corn kernels and return soup to boil. Simmer, uncovered, about 5 minutes longer.

5. Remove from heat and, using a ladle or slotted spoon, transfer about 2 1/2 cups of the vegetables to a blender or food processor. Puree until smooth.

6. Add puree and milk to saucepan and simmer about 3 minutes. Season with salt, pepper, and pinch of cayenne. Serve garnished with bacon.

Per cup: Calories: 88, fat: 3 g, saturated fat: 1 g, sodium: 87 mg, carbohydrate: 14 g, protein: 4 g.

Arugula Salad with Spicy Vinaigrette

This tart and refreshing side dish or appetizer has lots of vitamin C from the orange and its juice, the tomatoes, and even the greens. The arugula is also very high in calcium.

PREPARATION TIME: 25 MINUTES • **SERVES 4**

1/2	cup orange juice
2	tablespoons red wine vinegar
2	teaspoons jalapeño pepper sauce
1	teaspoon olive oil
1/2	teaspoon salt
1/4	teaspoon sugar
1/8	teaspoon pepper
8	cups arugula leaves
2	cups torn romaine lettuce
1	cup yellow and/or red cherry tomatoes, halved
1	navel orange, peeled and sliced into half-rounds
6	oil-cured black olives, slivered
1/2	small red onion, thinly sliced

1. In small bowl, whisk together orange juice, vinegar, jalapeño pepper sauce, oil, salt, sugar, and pepper.

2. In salad bowl, combine arugula, lettuce, tomatoes, orange, olives, and onion. Add dressing, tossing to coat well. Serve immediately.

Calories: 70, fat: 2 g, saturated fat: 0 g, sodium: 310 mg, carbohydrate: 13 g, protein: 3 g.

Bread Salad with Roasted Peppers

Red peppers have far more vitamin C than green peppers, making this a power dish for people with arthritis.

PREPARATION TIME: 15 MINUTES
COOKING TIME: 20 MINUTES • **SERVES 4**

4	large red bell peppers, cored and cut into flat panels
2	tablespoons balsamic vinegar
1	tablespoon olive oil
2	cups Italian or French bread cubes (1 inch)
3	large tomato, diced
1 1/2	cups diced cucumber
3	ounces feta cheese, crumbled
1/4	cup coarsely chopped kalamata, or other brine-cured olives

1. Preheat broiler. Place peppers, skin side up, on rack of broiling pan and broil 4 inches from heat for 12 minutes or until skin is blackened. Remove from broiler and allow to cool in brown paper bag. Peel cooled peppers and cut into 2-inch-wide strips.

2. In medium bowl, combine vinegar and oil. Add peppers and toss well. Refrigerate for at least 1 hour.

3. Preheat oven to 375°F. Spread bread cubes on baking sheet and bake, tossing occasionally, for 7 minutes or until lightly crisped, but not browned.

4. In large salad bowl, combine peppers and their marinade with toasted bread, tomato, cucumber, feta, and olives, tossing well. Serve at room temperature or chilled.

Calories: 340, fat: 13 g, saturated fat: 4 g, sodium: 750 mg, carbohydrate: 46 g, protein: 11 g.

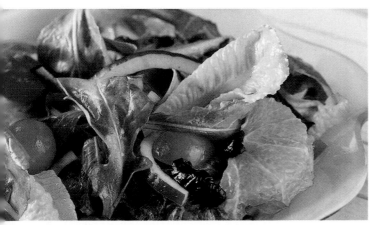

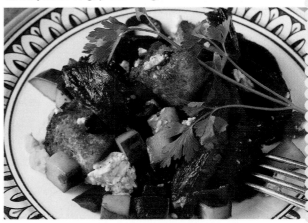

Crab & Grapefruit Salad

A summer treat that provides omega-3 fatty acids from the crab as well as lots of vitamin C from the grapefruit and calcium from the greens.

PREPARATION TIME: 25 MINUTES • **SERVES 4**

- 4 grapefruits
- 2 tablespoons light mayonnaise
- 1 tablespoon finely chopped mango chutney
- 2 teaspoons Dijon mustard
- 1 teaspoon sesame oil
- 1/4 teaspoon each salt and pepper
- 3/4 pound lump crabmeat, picked over to remove any cartilage
- 2 cups watercress, tough stems trimmed
- 1 Belgian endive, cut crosswise into 1/2-inch-wide strips
- 1 head Bibb lettuce, separated into leaves

1. With small paring knife, peel grapefruits. Working over bowl to catch juice, separate grapefruit sections from membranes; reserve juice that collects in bowl.

2. In medium bowl, whisk together mayonnaise, chutney, mustard, sesame oil, salt, pepper, and 3 tablespoons of reserved grapefruit juice.

3. Add crabmeat, tossing to combine. Add watercress, endive, and grapefruit sections, and toss. Serve salad on bed of Bibb lettuce.

Calories: 180, fat: 4 g, saturated fat: 1 g, sodium: 660 mg, carbohydrate: 20 g, protein: 18 g.

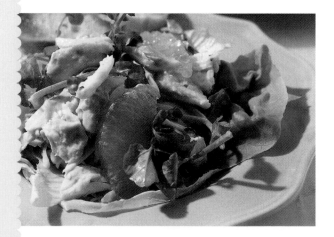

Cold Tuna & Vegetable Salad

This salad offers omega-3 fatty acids from the tuna and lots of vitamins C and B$_6$.

PREPARATION TIME: 45 MINUTES • **SERVES 4**

- 1 pound small red or white new potatoes
- 2 ounces (about 1 cup) thin green beans
- 2 large eggs
- 1/2 pound mixed lettuce leaves, washed
- 1 tablespoon chopped parsley
- 1 tablespoon snipped fresh chives
- 1 small red onion, sliced thin
- 1 tablespoon bottled tapenade (black olive paste)
- 2 garlic cloves, minced
- 2 tablespoons extra-virgin olive oil
- 1 tablespoon red wine vinegar
- 1 teaspoon balsamic vinegar
- 10–15 radishes, sliced thin
- 1 can (6 ounces) tuna packed in water, drained
- 1/2 cup cherry tomatoes
- 1 red bell pepper, seeded and sliced thin
- 1 yellow pepper, seeded and sliced thin
- 1 green pepper, seeded and sliced thin
- 8 black olives
  Fresh basil leaves, for garnish

1. Put potatoes in saucepan with water to cover and bring to boil. Simmer 10 minutes, add beans, and cook until vegetables are tender, 5 minutes more. Drain and rinse under cold water.

2. Put eggs in small saucepan with cold water to cover; bring to boil. Simmer gently for 5 minutes, drain, and rinse under cold water. Peel eggs and let stand in a bowl of cold water.

3. In large, shallow bowl, toss together lettuce, parsley, chives, and red onion.

4. In small bowl, whisk together tapenade, garlic, olive oil, vinegars, and salt and pepper to taste. Pour two-thirds of dressing over salad and toss.

5. Halve potatoes and arrange on top of salad with green beans, radishes, chunks of tuna, tomatoes, peppers, and olives. Quarter eggs and add to the salad. Pour remaining dressing on top and garnish with basil leaves.

Calories: 350, fat: 15 g, saturated fat: 3 g, sodium: 450 mg, carbohydrate: 36 g, protein: 18 g.

recipes for beating arthritis

Smoked Turkey & Melon Salad

Powerful portions of vitamins E and C star in this cool main-dish salad that takes the edge off hot weather.

PREPARATION TIME: 20 MINUTES • **SERVES 4**

3	cups honeydew and/or cantaloupe balls
3/4	pound smoked turkey breast, cut into 1/2-inch cubes
1/2	cup thinly sliced celery
2	scallions, sliced
2	tablespoons slivered fresh basil
2	tablespoons chopped toasted walnuts or pecans
2	tablespoons honey mustard
1	tablespoon white wine vinegar
2	teaspoons olive oil
1/2	teaspoon soy sauce

1. In large bowl, toss together melon balls, turkey, celery, scallions, basil, and walnuts.

2. In small bowl, whisk together honey mustard, vinegar, oil, and soy sauce. Toss dressing with melon mixture just before serving.

Calories: 210, fat: 8 g, saturated fat: 2 g, sodium: 850 mg, carbohydrate: 23 g, protein: 16 g.

Warm Snow Pea Salad with Mushrooms & Goat Cheese

Snow peas and watercress offer calcium and vitamin C, while mushrooms supply vitamin D. Red peppers give you more vitamin C and the goat cheese ups your total of calcium for this delectable salad. Pecans supply omega-3 fatty acids.

PREPARATION TIME: 15 MINUTES
COOKING TIME: 10 MINUTES
MARINATE: 20 MINUTES • **SERVES 4**

2	teaspoons olive oil
1/2	pound mushrooms, thinly sliced
2	cloves garlic, minced
1	pound snow peas, strings removed
1	small red bell pepper, cut into 2 x 1/4-inch strips
1/2	teaspoon salt
3	tablespoons rice vinegar
2	teaspoons honey
4	cups watercress leaves
4	ounces mild goat cheese
2	tablespoons pecans, toasted and chopped

1. In large nonstick skillet, over moderately high heat, heat 1 teaspoon of oil. Add mushrooms and sauté for 4 minutes or until tender and lightly browned. Add garlic and cook for 1 minute. Add snow peas, bell pepper, and salt, and sauté for 4 minutes or until crisp-tender.

2. Transfer to a large bowl and add vinegar, honey, and remaining 1 teaspoon oil, tossing to combine. Let stand for 20 minutes before serving.

3. Divide watercress among 4 salad plates and top with snow pea mixture. Sprinkle with goat cheese and pecans.

Calories: 240, fat: 14 g, saturated fat: 6 g, sodium: 400 mg, carbohydrate: 19 g, protein: 12 g.

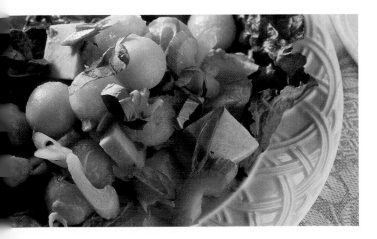

Grilled Steak & Vegetables

The vegetables offer up the main nutritional benefits—vitamin C, folate, and vitamin B₆—in this delightful barbecue. The canola oil adds omega-3 fatty acids, the beef adds more vitamin B₆, and the dish fits on a low-calorie diet.

PREPARATION TIME: 20 MINUTES PLUS MARINATING TIME
COOKING TIME: 20 MINUTES • **SERVES 4**

4	lean London broil steaks (4 ounces each)
3	tablespoons canola oil
3	tablespoons red wine vinegar
2	tablespoons Dijon mustard
2	cloves garlic, finely chopped
1	teaspoon each dried basil and oregano
1/8	teaspoon hot red pepper flakes
1/8	teaspoon each salt and freshly ground black pepper
2	sweet red or green peppers, cut lengthwise into 1-inch strips
3	zucchini, each cut lengthwise into 4 strips
2	red or yellow onions, cut across into 1/2-inch slices

1. Using a sharp knife, trim all fat from steaks.

2. Make marinade: In small bowl, combine oil with vinegar, mustard, garlic, basil, oregano, hot pepper flakes, salt, and pepper until blended.

3. Place steaks in dish just large enough to hold them and pour two-thirds of marinade over. Turn meat in marinade to coat it thoroughly. Cover dish and marinate in refrigerator at least 2 hours.

4. Remove meat from refrigerator and allow to come to room temperature. Pour off marinade and discard. Preheat a charcoal grill or broiler, setting rack 4 to 5 inches from the heat.

5. Add steaks to grill or broiler and cook according to taste, about 6 minutes on each side for medium. Meanwhile, using a small brush, coat vegetable pieces with remaining marinade mixture.

6. Transfer steaks to platter, cover with foil, and keep warm. Add the vegetables to grill or broiler and cook until browned and softened, turning once and brushing twice with the remaining marinade.

Calories: 327, fat: 18 g, saturated fat: 6 g, sodium: 271 mg, carbohydrate: 16 g, protein: 27 g.

Italian Beef & Broccoli Sauté

Broccoli, tomatoes, and peppers give this low-calorie dinner high marks for vitamin C. Broccoli adds plenty of calcium and the beef some vitamin B₆.

PREPARATION TIME: 25 MINUTES
COOKING TIME: 20 MINUTES • **SERVES 4**

3	pickled red cherry peppers
3/4	pound well-trimmed beef sirloin, thinly sliced
2	tablespoons balsamic vinegar
2	cloves garlic, minced
2	teaspoons olive oil
1	red onion, thinly sliced
1	yellow or red bell pepper, slivered
6	cups small broccoli florets
3/4	teaspoon dried oregano
2	cups cherry tomatoes, halved
1/3	cup chopped fresh basil
1/2	teaspoon salt

1. Mince one cherry pepper. In medium bowl, combine minced pepper, beef, vinegar, and garlic. Let stand for 15 minutes. Meanwhile, dice remaining cherry peppers.

2. In large skillet, heat oil over moderate heat. Add onion and bell pepper, and cook for 5 minutes. Add broccoli and oregano, reduce heat to moderately low, cover, and cook, stirring occasionally, for 10 minutes or until broccoli is crisp-tender.

3. Push vegetables to one side, increase heat to moderately high, and add reserved cherry peppers and beef with its marinade. Sauté for 2 minutes. Add cherry tomatoes, basil, and salt, and sauté for 2 minutes or until heated through.

Calories: 280, fat: 12 g, saturated fat: 4 g, sodium: 330 mg, carbohydrate: 17 g, protein: 29 g.

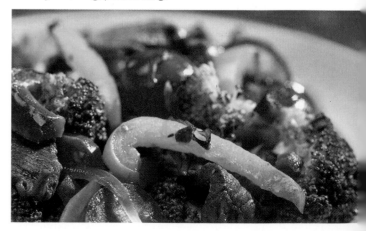

Spicy Lamb Stew with Couscous

Capture the atmosphere of Morocco with this vitamin-filled stew, called a tagine, in which zucchini, carrots, tomatoes, onions, and apricots all contribute vitamin C and several contribute folate and/or vitamin E.

PREPARATION TIME: 35 MINUTES
COOKING TIME: 2 HOURS • **SERVES 6**

1 3/4	pounds boneless leg of lamb, trimmed and cut into 1-inch cubes
1	small onion, chopped
2	cloves garlic, chopped
1/2	teaspoon cayenne pepper
1	cinnamon stick, broken in half
1	teaspoon ground ginger
1	teaspoon sweet paprika
1/4	teaspoon crumbled saffron threads
3/4	cup dried apricots, quartered
1	cup chopped carrots
1	cup chopped zucchini
2	medium tomatoes, chopped
3	tablespoons chopped fresh coriander
3	tablespoons chopped fresh parsley
1 1/2	cups (about 10 ounces) couscous

1. In a large saucepan, combine lamb, onion, garlic, cayenne pepper, cinnamon, ginger, paprika, saffron, and salt and pepper to taste. Add enough water to cover and simmer mixture, covered, for 1 hour 30 minutes.

2. Add apricots, carrots, zucchini, tomatoes, 2 tablespoons coriander and 2 tablespoons parsley to pan and simmer, covered, 15 minutes more.

3. Meanwhile, put couscous in a bowl, add just enough cold water to cover it and let it stand for 5 minutes to absorb the liquid.

4. Transfer couscous to a sieve, and steam couscous over stew until warm, about 15 minutes. Fluff with fork and add salt to taste.

5. To serve, spoon couscous onto serving dish. Using a slotted spoon, top couscous with lamb and vegetables and sprinkle with remaining coriander and parsley. Serve cooking liquid on side as a sauce.

Calories: 420, fat: 7 g, saturated fat: 2 g, sodium: 100 mg, carbohydrate: 54 g, protein: 35 g.

Lamb Curry

In this mild curry, lean lamb gives you vitamin B_6 and folate; the yogurt gives calcium; the onions and tomato paste give vitamins C, E, and folate.

PREPARATION TIME: 35 MINUTES
COOKING TIME: 1 HOUR 10 MINUTES • **SERVES 4**

1/3	cup plain low-fat yogurt
1/2	teaspoon cayenne pepper
2	teaspoons ground coriander
1 1/2	teaspoons ground cumin
2	teaspoons crushed garlic
2	teaspoons grated fresh ginger
1	teaspoon sweet paprika
1/2	teaspoon ground turmeric
1 1/4	pounds boneless leg of lamb, trimmed and cut into 2-inch cubes
1 3/4	cups finely chopped onion
1 1/2	tablespoons tomato paste
	Salt to taste
2	tablespoons unsalted butter
2	bay leaves
2	green cardamom pods, tops split open
1	cinnamon stick, broken in half
4	whole cloves
1/2	teaspoon freshly grated nutmeg
1	tablespoon chopped fresh mint
2	tablespoons chopped fresh coriander

1. In small bowl, combine first 8 ingredients.

2. In nonstick saucepan, medium heat, cook lamb and onions, stirring until meat begins to sizzle.

3. Add yogurt mixture. Over low heat, cook, covered, stirring occasionally, until lamb releases its juices, about 30 minutes. Cook uncovered, medium heat, stirring frequently, until sauce reduces to pastelike consistency, 5–6 minutes.

4. Stir in tomato paste, salt, and 1 tablespoon butter. Reduce heat to low and cook, uncovered, for 3 minutes, stirring frequently. Stir in 3/4 cup boiling water and simmer, covered, for 15 minutes.

5. In small skillet, low heat, melt 1 tablespoon butter. Add bay leaves, cardamom, cinnamon and cloves and sizzle for 35–40 seconds. Add nutmeg, stir once; pour over meat. Stir well and simmer, covered, 10 minutes. Stir in mint and coriander.

Calories: 300, fat: 13 g, saturated fat: 6 g, sodium: 135 mg, carbohydrate: 12 g, protein: 32 g.

Mediterranean Lamb Roast & Potatoes

This one-dish meal is an easy Greek-style roast bursting with the fresh flavors of lemon and herbs and offering an array of arthritis-healthy nutrients. You will get vitamin B$_6$ and folate from the lamb, vitamins C and E from the tomatoes, vitamin C and folate from the onions or shallots, vitamins B$_6$ and C from the potatoes, and vitamin C from the lemon.

PREPARATION TIME: 15–20 MINUTES **COOKING TIME:** 1 HOUR–1 HOUR, 5 MINUTES • **SERVES 4**

1 1/4	pounds boneless leg of lamb, trimmed and cut into 1-inch cubes
2	medium onions, cut into quarters, or 3/4 pound shallots, peeled but left whole
1 1/4	pounds small new potatoes, scrubbed and halved if large
1	large lemon, cut into 8 wedges
1	tablespoon olive oil
12	garlic cloves, peeled
6	sprigs fresh rosemary
6	sprigs fresh thyme
1/3	pound cherry or grape tomatoes, halved
1	tablespoon bottled mint sauce, or 2 tablespoons mint jelly, melted

1. Preheat oven to 400°F.

2. Arrange lamb, onions or shallots, and potatoes in a large roasting pan. Squeeze juice from four lemon wedges over meat and vegetables and drizzle with oil. Tuck all eight lemon wedges, garlic, and half of herbs among meat and vegetables and season with salt and pepper. Cover tightly with foil and roast for 45 minutes.

3. Remove pan from oven, discard foil and herbs, and increase oven to 425°F. Add tomatoes, remaining herbs and mint sauce or jelly and toss meat and vegetables well. Roast, uncovered, until meat and vegetables are browned and tender, 15 to 20 minutes.

Calories: 420, fat: 10 g, saturated fat: 3 g, sodium: 105 mg, carbohydrate: 49 g, protein: 34 g.

Spinach-Stuffed Meat Loaf

Spinach is a superfood for people with arthritis—with vitamins B$_6$, C, E, folate, and calcium. Beef and turkey add to the vitamin B$_6$. Ricotta shores you up with calcium, and the onions, tomatoes, and carrots together give you lots of vitamin C and some vitamin E and folate.

PREPARATION TIME: 30 MINUTES
COOKING TIME: 11/2 HOURS • **SERVES 6**

1	pound lean ground beef
8	ounces lean ground turkey
1	small onion, finely chopped
1/2	cup fresh bread crumbs
1/8	teaspoon garlic salt
1	tablespoon tomato paste
1	egg white
1/2	cup part-skim ricotta cheese
1	package (10 ounces) frozen chopped spinach, thawed and drained
1/8	teaspoon each salt and pepper
2	large onions, thinly sliced
2	carrots, coarsely chopped
1	can (28 ounces) crushed tomatoes

1. In a bowl, mix beef, turkey, chopped onion, bread crumbs, garlic salt, and tomato paste. In another bowl, mix egg white, ricotta, spinach, salt, and pepper.

2. Preheat oven to 350°F. Turn out beef mixture onto a large sheet of wax paper, and form into a 9"x10" rectangle with your hands.

3. Spoon spinach stuffing lengthwise down center of meat, leaving about 1 inch uncovered at each short end.

4. With help of wax paper, lift long edges of meat. Fold meat over stuffing to enclose it.

5. Using your fingers, pinch edges of meat together. Place loaf seam side down in a nonstick roasting pan. Add onions, carrots, and tomatoes to pan.

6. Bake about 11/2 hours or until meat and vegetables are cooked. Transfer meat to platter. Puree vegetables in a blender and serve sauce with meat loaf.

Calories: 294, fat: 6 g, saturated fat: 2 g, sodium: 405 mg, carbohydrate: 28 g, protein: 32 g.

Beef & Turkey Chili

Both beef and turkey provide you with vitamin B₆; the kidney beans are a prime source of folate; the tomatoes give you vitamins C and E; the onions, peppers, and corn give you more vitamin C and folate. That makes for a hearty and healthy chili!

PREPARATION TIME: 20 MINUTES
COOKING TIME: 50–60 MINUTES • **SERVES 6**

1	pound lean ground beef
8	ounces lean ground turkey
1	tablespoon canola oil
2	large onions, coarsely chopped
3	cloves garlic, finely chopped
3	sweet red or green peppers, coarsely chopped
1	tablespoon chili powder or more to taste
1	teaspoon each ground cumin and coriander
1	can (28 ounces) crushed tomatoes
	Dash of hot red pepper sauce (optional)
1/8	teaspoon pepper
1	package (10 ounces) frozen corn kernels, thawed
1	can (16 ounces) red kidney beans, drained and rinsed

1. Heat a Dutch oven over moderately high heat until hot. Add beef and turkey and sauté, stirring frequently, about 7 minutes or until meat has lost its pink color and has released its juices.

2. Remove from heat and spoon meat into a sieve set over a bowl. Allow all fat to drain from meat; it will take at least 10 minutes.

3. Meanwhile, in Dutch oven, heat oil over moderate heat. Add onions and garlic and sauté 5 to 7 minutes or until softened and golden brown.

4. Stir in sweet peppers, chili powder, and spices and cook about 5 minutes longer or until peppers are slightly soft. Return meat to Dutch oven.

5. Stir in crushed tomatoes, hot pepper sauce, if using, and pepper and bring to a boil. Partially cover and simmer, stirring occasionally, 20 to 30 minutes or until sauce thickens.

6. Stir in corn kernels and kidney beans. Cover and cook about 5 minutes longer to heat through.

Calories: 340, fat: 7 g, saturated fat: 2 g, sodium: 546 mg, carbohydrate: 37 g, protein: 34 g.

Chicken Stew with Balsamic Vinegar

Balsamic vinegar brings a new twist to a classic!

PREPARATION TIME: 15 MINUTES
COOKING TIME: 40 MINUTES • **SERVES 4**

1	slice thick-cut bacon (2 ounces)
1	broiler-fryer (2 1/2 to 3 pounds), skinned and cut into serving-size pieces
1/4	teaspoon each salt and black pepper
1	package (10 ounces) frozen pearl onions
8	ounces small mushrooms, quartered
1/4	cup balsamic vinegar
1/2	cup dry red wine
1 1/2	cups chicken stock
1	can (14 1/2 ounces) low-sodium tomatoes, drained and chopped
1	teaspoon each dried rosemary and thyme, crumbled
1	tablespoon arrowroot or cornstarch mixed with 2 tablespoons water
2	tablespoons minced fresh parsley

1. In 12-inch nonstick skillet, cook bacon over moderate heat for 2 minutes or until crisp. Drain bacon on paper towels, then crumble and set aside. Discard all but 1 tablespoon fat in skillet. Sprinkle chicken with 1/8 teaspoon each salt and pepper. Set skillet over moderate heat; when bacon fat is hot, sauté chicken on each side until lightly browned, 2 minutes. Transfer chicken to 5-quart Dutch oven.

2. Add onions, mushrooms, and remaining salt and pepper to skillet and sauté, stirring occasionally, for 5 minutes. Transfer vegetables to a bowl. Add vinegar and wine to skillet; bring to boil over moderately high heat. Boil mixture, stirring, for 1 minute; add to Dutch oven with chicken.

3. Add stock, tomatoes, rosemary, and thyme to Dutch oven; bring to a boil. Cover, simmer over low heat until the breast meat is no longer pink inside, 15 minutes. Transfer breast pieces to plate; add onions and mushrooms to Dutch oven. Cover, simmer until onions are tender and juices run clear, 8–10 minutes more.

4. Return breast pieces to Dutch oven and bring liquid to a boil. Stir in arrowroot mixture and simmer over low heat for 2 to 3 minutes or until the sauce has thickened. Sprinkle with tarragon.

Calories: 380, fat: 13 g, saturated fat: 4 g, sodium: 578 mg, carbohydrate: 16 g, protein: 45 g.

Grilled Chicken with Herbs

A tasty chicken that gives you vitamin B_6 is marinated in canola oil, with its omega-3 fatty acids, and herbs to give the chicken a lovely flavor.

PREPARATION TIME: 15 MINUTES
COOKING TIME: 30 MINUTES
MARINATE: 4 HOURS • **SERVES 4**

1	chicken (about 3 1/2 pounds), cut into serving pieces, wings reserved for another use
3	cloves garlic, finely chopped
3	tablespoons chopped parsley
2	tablespoons chopped basil
2	tablespoons chopped mint
1/3	cup canola oil
1/2	teaspoon pepper
1/8	teaspoon salt

1. Loosen skin of chicken with tip of a sharp knife, then pull it off. Cut off any fat and make 2 to 3 slashes in each piece of chicken.

2. Make marinade: In a small bowl, combine garlic with parsley, basil, mint, oil, pepper, and salt.

3. Place chicken in large dish, add marinade, and coat chicken well. Cover and marinate in refrigerator at least 4 hours, turning chicken occasionally.

4. Prepare grill or preheat broiler, setting rack 4 inches from heat. Arrange chicken pieces bone side down on grill or broiler rack, reserving marinade. Grill chicken about 20 minutes or until browned on one side, brushing once with reserved marinade. Turn pieces over, brush with remaining marinade, and grill 10 minutes longer or until cooked through and juices run clear.

Calories: 306, fat: 15 g, saturated fat: 3 g, sodium: 208 mg, carbohydrate: 2g, protein: 40 g.

Spicy Asian Chicken Braised with Mushrooms

Hoisin sauce, sold in jars in the Asian foods section of the supermarket, is made from soybeans, garlic, chiles, and other seasonings. It's a potent source of vitamin E and calcium. Mushrooms will give you vitamin D, which helps your body absorb calcium. Rounding out the benefits of this dish are the chicken pieces that give you vitamin B_6 and the peppers that give you B_6, C, and folate.

PREPARATION TIME: 15 MINUTES
COOKING TIME: 40 MINUTES • **SERVES 4**

3	scallions, thinly sliced
3	cloves garlic, crushed and peeled
3	slices (1/4-inch-thick) fresh ginger
1/4	cup lower-sodium soy sauce
1/4	cup hoisin sauce
1/4	cup chicken broth
1	tablespoon sesame oil
1	teaspoon crushed red pepper flakes
1	teaspoon sugar
3/4	teaspoon salt
8	chicken drumsticks (about 2 1/2 pounds), skin removed
1	pound mushrooms, quartered
1	large green bell pepper, cut into 1/2-inch pieces
1 1/2	teaspoons cornstarch blended with 1 tablespoon water
1	cup rice

1. In Dutch oven, stir together scallions, garlic, ginger, soy sauce, hoisin sauce, broth, sesame oil, red pepper flakes, sugar, and 1/4 teaspoon of salt. Stir in chicken, mushrooms, and bell pepper.

2. Bring to a boil over medium heat. Reduce heat to a simmer, cover, and cook 35 minutes or until chicken is cooked through and vegetables are tender. Stir in cornstarch mixture and cook, stirring constantly, for 1 minute or until slightly thickened.

3. Meanwhile, in medium covered saucepan, bring 21/4 cups of water to a boil. Add rice and remaining 1/2 teaspoon salt. Reduce heat to a simmer, cover, and cook 17 minutes or until rice is tender. Serve sauce and chicken with rice.

Calories: 490, fat: 10 g, saturated fat: 2 g, sodium: 1561 mg, carbohydrate: 58 g, protein: 39 g.

Pesto Chicken on Focaccia

In Italy, a slice of focaccia is a popular snack. When you add vitamin B$_6$-rich chicken to this thick slice of bread, along with calcium-rich cheese, vitamin E-rich nuts, and peppers with their vitamins B$_6$ and C, as well as folate, you are talking serious good nutrition for someone with arthritis.

PREPARATION TIME: 15 MINUTES, **COOKING TIME:** 15 MINUTES • **SERVES 4**

1	clove garlic, peeled
1/2	cup packed fresh basil leaves
3	tablespoons grated Parmesan cheese
1	tablespoon plus 2 teaspoons olive oil
2	tablespoons slivered almonds
1/4	teaspoon salt
1	round focaccia (10-inch diameter, 8 ounces)
2	cups mixed greens
2	cooked skinless, boneless chicken breast halves (leftover or poached), thinly sliced crosswise on the diagonal
1/2	cup bottled roasted red peppers, cut into thin strips

1. Preheat oven to 400°F. To make the pesto: In small pan of boiling water, blanch garlic 1 minute. Drain and transfer to food processor. Add basil, Parmesan, oil, almonds, salt, and 2 tablespoons of water, and process until smooth.

2. Bake focaccia for 10 minutes. When cool enough to handle, slice in half horizontally. Spread pesto onto both focaccia halves. Top with mixed greens. Place chicken and then roasted peppers on top of greens. Cover with focaccia top. To serve, cut into 4 wedges.

Calories: 356, fat: 13 g, saturated fat: 3 g, sodium: 599 mg, carbohydrate: 30 g, protein: 30 g.

Poached Chicken

This simple recipe covers quite a few nutritional bases: The chicken gives you vitamin B$_6$; the carrots give you vitamin C; the potatoes give you a little more of each. Plus, the leeks and lemon juice add to the vitamin C count.

PREPARATION TIME: 25–30 MINUTES **COOKING TIME:** 1 1/4–1 1/2 HOURS, MOSTLY UNATTENDED • **SERVES 4**

1	whole chicken (3 1/2 pounds)
6	cups chicken stock
5	cups water
4	carrots, cut into 1-inch pieces
2	leeks, white part only, sliced
2	large potatoes, peeled and cut into cubes
6	cloves garlic, peeled
1	bouquet garni, made with 8 sprigs parsley and 2 bay leaves
1	tablespoon lemon juice
1/8	teaspoon each salt and pepper

1. Cut fat from both ends of bird and wipe inside with paper towels. Tuck wings under bird. Fold skin over body cavity opening; tie legs together with string.

2. Place chicken in a 4-quart Dutch oven. Add stock and water to cover. Bring to a boil over moderate heat and, using a large spoon, skim off any scum.

3. Add vegetables, garlic, and herbs to Dutch oven and simmer, partially covered, about 1 1/4 hours or until chicken and vegetables are cooked through.

4. Transfer chicken to a platter, cover with aluminum foil, and keep warm. Strain stock into a bowl and skim off fat. Reserve vegetables and discard herbs.

5. In a blender or food processor, puree half of vegetables and 1 1/2 cups stock; pour into a pan. Add lemon juice, salt, and pepper.

6. Remove skin from chicken and carve meat. Meanwhile, warm sauce gently. Place chicken and remaining vegetables on a platter and pour sauce over.

Calories: 299, fat: 7 g, saturated fat: 2 g, sodium: 354 mg, carbohydrate: 30 g, protein: 47 g.

Sesame Chicken Salad

The perfect summer entrée, this Chinese-style chicken and vegetable salad offers plenty of calcium from snow peas, vitamin C from peppers and snow peas, and vitamin B$_6$ from snow peas and chicken.

PREPARATION TIME: 20 MINUTE,
COOKING TIME: 2 MINUTES • **SERVES 4**

2	cloves garlic, peeled
1/2	pound snow peas, strings removed
1	red bell pepper, cut into 2-inch-long matchsticks
1	piece (2 inches) fresh ginger, peeled and thickly sliced
3	tablespoons sesame oil
3	tablespoons lower-sodium soy sauce
2 1/2	teaspoons sugar
2 1/2	teaspoons rice vinegar
1/4	teaspoon crushed red pepper flakes
1	cucumber, peeled, halved lengthwise, seeded, and cut into 2-inch-long matchsticks
2	cups shredded cooked chicken breasts or thighs—leftover or poached

1. In large pot of boiling water, blanch garlic 1 minute; remove with slotted spoon. Add snow peas and bell pepper, and blanch 15 seconds; drain well.

2. In food processor, combine blanched garlic, ginger, sesame oil, soy sauce, sugar, vinegar, and red pepper flakes, and process until smooth.

3. Transfer dressing to large bowl. Add snow peas, bell pepper, cucumber, and chicken, and toss to combine. Serve at room temperature or chilled.

Calories: 263, fat: 13 g, saturated fat: 2 g, sodium: 508 mg, carbohydrate: 12 g, protein: 25 g.

Thai Chicken Stew

Thai cooking demands a careful balance of tastes and textures. There is also a balance of nutrients: vitamin E and calcium from the soy milk; vitamin B$_6$ from the chicken, bell pepper, potatoes, and peanut butter; vitamin C from the bell pepper, potatoes, and lime juice, and folate from the peanut butter.

PREPARATION TIME: 25 MINUTES
COOKING TIME: 20 MINUTES • **SERVES 4**

2	teaspoons vegetable oil
1	red bell pepper, cut into 1/2-inch squares
2	cloves garlic, minced
1	tablespoon minced fresh ginger
3/4	pound all-purpose potatoes (2 to 3 medium), peeled and cut into 1/2-inch chunks
1	cup chicken broth
1	pound skinless, boneless chicken breasts, cut into 1-inch chunks
2	cups unflavored soy milk
1/3	cup chopped fresh basil
1/4	cup chopped cilantro
2	tablespoons lime juice
2	tablespoons lower-sodium soy sauce
1	tablespoon reduced-fat peanut butter
2	teaspoons dark brown sugar
1/4	teaspoon coconut extract

1. In large nonstick skillet, heat oil over moderate heat. Add bell pepper, garlic, and ginger, and sauté for 4 minutes or until pepper is crisp-tender. Add potatoes and broth, and bring to a boil. Reduce to a simmer, cover, and cook for 7 minutes or until potatoes are firm-tender.

2. Add chicken, soy milk, basil, cilantro, lime juice, soy sauce, peanut butter, brown sugar, and coconut extract to pan, and bring to a boil. Reduce to a simmer, cover, and cook for 5 minutes or until chicken and potatoes are cooked through.

Calories: 430, fat: 21 g, saturated fat: 6 g, sodium: 410 mg, carbohydrate: 34 g, protein: 27 g.

Turkey Quesadillas

This spicy Southwestern dish can also be made with ground chicken, beef, or pork, which give you vitamin B$_6$ just like the turkey. The peppers and onions offer vitamin C and folate, and the cheese provides calcium.

PREPARATION TIME: 20 MINUTES
COOKING TIME: 25 MINUTES • **SERVES 6**

6	flour tortillas, 7 inches in diameter
2	teaspoons olive oil
1	medium yellow onion, finely chopped (1 cup)
1	medium sweet red pepper, cored, seeded, and diced (3/4 cup)
1 1/4	pounds ground turkey
1/4	teaspoon salt
2	cloves garlic, minced
1	teaspoon each ground cumin, chili powder, and dried oregano, crumbled
1	jalapeño pepper, seeded and finely chopped (1 tablespoon)
1/2	cup low-sodium tomato sauce
2	tablespoons minced fresh cilantro (coriander) or 2 tablespoons minced parsley mixed with 3/4 teaspoon dried cilantro
1/2	cup grated Monterey Jack cheese (2 ounces)
1	cup tomato salsa (optional)

1. Preheat oven to 350°F. Wrap tortillas in aluminum foil and heat in oven for 8 minutes. Meanwhile, in 12-inch nonstick skillet, heat oil over moderate heat. Add onion and red pepper and sauté, stirring occasionally, for 5 minutes or until onion is soft.

2. Add turkey and salt to skillet and sauté, stirring, for 3 minutes or until turkey is no longer pink. Add garlic, cumin, chili powder, oregano, and jalapeño pepper; sauté, stirring, for 1 minute or until mixture is dry. Stir in tomato sauce and cilantro.

3. Increase oven temperature to 450°F. Unwrap tortillas and place on greased baking sheets. Spread equal amount of turkey mixture on each one and sprinkle with cheese. Bake for 8 to 10 minutes or until cheese is melted and tortillas are golden. Serve with salsa if desired.

Calories: 277, fat: 9 g, saturated fat: 1 g, sodium: 213 mg, carbohydrate: 22 g, protein: 26 g.

Salmon Steaks Mexican-Style

A healthy, and delicious, supplier of omega-3 fatty acids, salmon gets a spicy treatment in this recipe, which also offers lots of vitamin C (tomatoes, onions, lime juice, hot pepper), a little vitamin E (tomatoes), and folate (onions and pepper).

PREPARATION TIME: 15 MINUTES
COOKING TIME: 55 MINUTES • **SERVES 4**

2	teaspoons olive oil
1	small onion, finely chopped
2	cloves garlic, minced
1	teaspoon chili powder
1	can (14 1/2 ounces) no-salt-added tomatoes, chopped, with their juice
1	pickled jalapeño, finely chopped
1/4	cup pitted green olives, coarsely chopped
1 1/2	teaspoons capers, rinsed and drained
1/4	teaspoon each dried oregano and thyme
1/8	teaspoon each cinnamon and salt
4	salmon steaks (8 ounces each)
2	tablespoons lime juice

1. In a large nonstick skillet, heat oil over moderate heat. Sauté onion and garlic until soft, 5 minutes. Add chili powder, stirring to coat onions. Add tomatoes, jalapeño, olives, capers, oregano, thyme, cinnamon, salt, and 1/4 cup water; bring to a boil. Reduce heat, cover, and simmer until sauce is richly flavored, 30 minutes.

2. Preheat oven to 350°F. Sprinkle salmon with lime juice; place in 9" x 13" baking dish. Spoon 3/4 cup sauce over fish and bake until it flakes when tested with a fork, 15–20 minutes. Reheat remaining sauce; spoon over fish.

Calories: 500, fat: 29 g, saturated fat: 5 g, sodium: 530 mg, carbohydrate: 12 g, protein: 46 g.

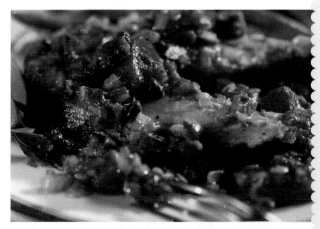

Broiled Herb-Rubbed Salmon

This simple and speedy way of cooking salmon brings out all its good flavor and gives you a full shot of omega-3 fatty acids.

PREPARATION TIME: 10 MINUTES
COOKING TIME: 5 MINUTES • **SERVES 4**

3/4	teaspoon salt
1/2	teaspoon sugar
1/2	teaspoon crumbled dried rosemary
1/4	teaspoon dried tarragon
	Pinch ground allspice
4	six-ounce salmon fillets

1. Preheat broiler. In small bowl, combine salt, sugar, rosemary, tarragon, and ground allspice.

2. Rub mixture into salmon fillets.

3. Broil, skin side down, 6 inches from heat, without turning, for 5 minutes or until salmon just flakes when tested with a fork.

Calories: 310, fat: 18 g, saturated fat: 4 g, sodium: 450 mg, carbohydrate: 1 g, protein: 34 g.

Summer Salmon & Asparagus

Fresh young vegetables and succulent salmon make this casserole highly nutritious—in addition to the omega-3 fatty acids supplied by the fish, you gain vitamin C and folate from the leeks, and vitamins C and B$_6$ and folate from the asparagus.

PREPARATION TIME: 10 MINUTES
COOKING TIME: ABOUT 20 MINUTES • **SERVES 4**

4	skinless salmon fillets, about 5 ounces each
7	ounces baby leeks
8	ounces tender asparagus spears
5	ounces sugar snap peas
4	tablespoons dry white wine
3/4	cup fish or vegetable stock, preferably fresh stock
2	tablespoons butter, diced
	Salt and fresh-ground black pepper
1	tablespoon snipped fresh chives

1. Run your fingertips over each salmon fillet to check for stray bones, pulling out any that you find. In bottom of a large, shallow flameproof casserole, arrange leeks in a single layer. Lay salmon fillets on top. Surround fish with asparagus and sugar snap peas. Pour in wine and stock, and dot fish with butter. Season with salt and pepper to taste.

2. Bring to a boil, then cover casserole with tight-fitting lid and reduce heat so liquid simmers gently. Simmer fish and vegetables until salmon is pale pink all the way through and vegetables are fork-tender, 12 to 14 minutes. Sprinkle chives over salmon.

Calories: 370, fat: 21 g, saturated fat: 7 g, sodium: 220 mg, carbohydrate: 9 g, protein: 33 g.

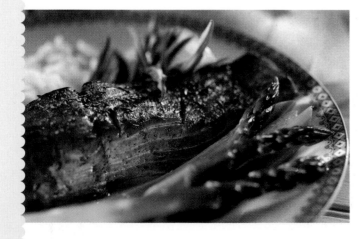

Walnut-Crusted Snapper

Walnuts have vitamin E; snapper fillets, omega-3 fatty acids; lemon juice and zest, vitamin C; and Parmesan, plenty of calcium. This is a terrific low-calorie dinner entrée for watching your weight and your arthritis.

PREPARATION TIME: 10 MINUTES
COOKING TIME: 15 MINUTES • **SERVES 4**

3	tablespoons light mayonnaise
1/2	teaspoon grated lemon zest
1	teaspoon lemon juice
1/4	teaspoon each salt and pepper
4	red snapper fillets (6 ounces each), skinned
1/2	cup walnut halves
2	tablespoons grated Parmesan cheese

1. Preheat oven to 450°F. Spray a large baking sheet with nonstick cooking spray; set aside.

2. In a small bowl, combine mayonnaise, lemon zest, lemon juice, salt, and pepper. Place fillets, skinned side down, on prepared baking sheet. Spread mayonnaise mixture over fish.

3. In food processor, process walnuts and Parmesan until finely ground (but not pasty). Sprinkle nut mixture over fish, patting it on. Bake for 15 minutes or until nuts are lightly browned and fish is just cooked through or just flakes when tested with a fork.

Calories: 320, fat: 16 g, saturated fat: 2 g, sodium: 370 mg, carbohydrate: 3 g, protein: 40 g.

Garlic, Tomato, & Anchovy Toasts

Anchovies give these toasts a sharp, salty taste along with omega-3 fatty acids. The tomatoes and lemon juice add a healthy shot of vitamin C.

PREPARATION TIME: 5 MINUTES, PLUS 10 MINUTES SOAKING
COOKING TIME: 2–3 MINUTES • **SERVES 4**

3	anchovy fillets
2	tablespoons skim milk
1	clove garlic, crushed
1	teaspoon fresh lemon juice
4	diagonal slices of Italian or French bread, 1 inch thick
2	tomatoes, sliced thin
1	tablespoon olive oil
	Freshly ground black pepper
1/4	cup small basil leaves

1. In a small dish, soak anchovies in milk for 10 minutes. Drain, rinse, and pat fish dry. Mash anchovies, garlic, and lemon juice with a mortar and pestle or a fork until they form a paste.

2. Preheat broiler with rack set 6 inches from heat. Toast bread on both sides under broiler. Spread one fourth of paste thinly on one side of each slice.

3. Arrange tomato slices on top of toasts. Drizzle with oil, season with pepper and place on baking sheet. Broil until tomatoes are softened, 1 to 2 minutes. Top with basil.

Calories: 180, fat: 5 g, saturated fat: 2 g, sodium: 290 mg, carbohydrate: 27 g, protein: 6 g.

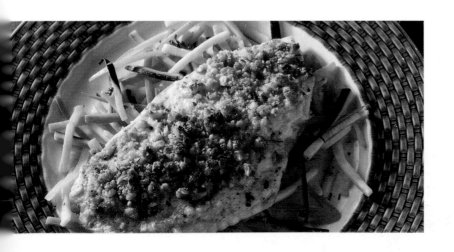

Grilled Halibut Steaks with Tomato & Red Pepper Salsa

Fish steaks make healthy fast food. In 20 minutes you can have a good supply of omega-3 fatty acids from the fish and vitamins C, B$_6$, and E as well as folate from the salsa.

PREPARATION TIME: 15 MINUTES
COOKING TIME: 4–6 MINUTES • **SERVES 4**

4	small halibut steaks
3	tablespoons extra-virgin olive oil
	Juice of 1 small orange
1	garlic clove, crushed

For salsa:

1/2	pound plum tomatoes, diced
1/2	red bell pepper, seeded and diced
1/2	red onion, chopped fine
	Juice of 1 small orange
1/4	cup chopped fresh basil
1	tablespoon balsamic vinegar
1	teaspoon sugar
	Orange wedges for garnish

1. Place halibut steaks in shallow baking dish. In small bowl, stir together oil, orange juice, garlic, and salt and pepper to taste. Spoon over fish.

2. In serving bowl, combine the salsa ingredients with salt and pepper to taste and let stand at room temperature.

3. Heat a lightly oiled ridged cast-iron grill pan or heavy-based frying pan over a high heat. Cook fish steaks for 2–3 minutes on each side, basting occasionally with the oil mixture, until fish just flakes.

4. Serve fish with salsa.

Calories: 270, fat: 13 g, saturated fat: 2 g, sodium: 70 mg, carbohydrate: 11 g, protein: 25 g.

Asian Stuffed Shrimp Salad

Shrimp is a rich source of omega-3 fatty acids; the vegetables add vitamin C and folate.

PREPARATION TIME: 30 MINUTES
COOKING TIME: 10 MINUTES • **SERVES 4**

16	jumbo shrimp (1 1/2 pounds), peeled and deveined
1/3	cup chopped cilantro
1	clove garlic, minced
1	tablespoon olive oil
2	carrots, julienned
2	scallions, cut into 2 x 1/4-inch strips
1	tablespoon minced fresh ginger
2	tablespoons lower-sodium soy sauce
2	tablespoons chili sauce
4	teaspoons lime juice
1	teaspoon sugar
6	cups torn romaine lettuce leaves
1	cucumber, peeled, halved lengthwise, seeded, and sliced
2	tablespoons chopped fresh mint

1. With paring knife, cut along back of shrimp until you have cut almost, but not quite through, to other side. In a large bowl, toss together shrimp, cilantro, garlic, and 1 teaspoon of oil; set aside.

2. In large nonstick skillet, heat remaining 2 teaspoons oil over moderate heat. Add carrots and scallions, and sauté for 2 minutes. Add ginger and cook for 2 minutes. Cool vegetable mixture to room temperature.

3. Preheat broiler. Place shrimp, cut side up, on a broiler pan, pressing down to flatten shrimp slightly. Spoon vegetable mixture onto shrimp and broil 6 inches from heat for 4 minutes or until shrimp are just cooked through.

4. Meanwhile, in a large bowl, combine soy sauce, chili sauce, lime juice, and sugar. Add lettuce, cucumber, and mint, tossing to combine. Serve shrimp on a bed of the salad mixture.

Calories: 240, fat: 6 g, saturated fat: 1 g, sodium: 680 mg, carbohydrate: 9 g, protein: 38 g.

French Shrimp Stew

Seafood stews from the Mediterranean basin are frequently accented with the licorice-like taste of fennel, a prime source of vitamin C. In this aromatic dish, you will also get omega-3 fatty acids from the shrimp and more vitamin C from the tomatoes, peppers, and onions, as well as some folate and vitamins E and B$_6$.

PREPARATION TIME: 30 MINUTES
COOKING TIME: 35 MINUTES • **SERVES 4**

1	red bell pepper, cut lengthwise into flat panels
1/2	teaspoon hot pepper sauce
1	tablespoon olive oil
1	small onion, finely chopped
2	cloves garlic, minced
1	small bulb fennel, trimmed and cut into 1/2-inch pieces
2/3	cup canned no-salt-added tomatoes, chopped with their juice
1/2	cup chicken broth
3/4	teaspoon grated orange zest
1/2	teaspoon salt
1	pound medium shrimp, peeled and deveined
4	slices French or Italian bread, toasted

1. Preheat broiler. Place bell pepper pieces, skin side up, on the broiler rack and broil 4 inches from heat for 12 minutes or until skin is blackened. Place in paper bag to cool and then peel and transfer to a food processor or blender. Add hot pepper sauce and 1 teaspoon oil, and puree.

2. Meanwhile, in large nonstick skillet, heat remaining 2 teaspoons oil over moderate heat. Add onion and garlic, and sauté for 5 minutes or until soft. Add fennel, and cook for 7 minutes or until tender. Stir in tomatoes, broth, orange zest, and salt. Bring to a boil, reduce to a simmer, cover, and cook for 5 minutes.

3. Add shrimp to skillet and cook for 4 minutes or until just cooked through. Stir roasted pepper puree into skillet. Serve stew with toast.

Calories: 220, fat: 5 g, saturated fat: 1 g, sodium: 730 mg, carbohydrate: 15 g, protein: 26 g.

Penne with Sugar Snaps & Smoked Salmon

This is a pasta dish that gives you omega-3 fatty acids from the salmon, vitamin C from the lemon juice and zest, calcium and vitamin C from the sugar snap peas, and vitamin C and folate from the scallions.

PREPARATION TIME: 20 MINUTES
COOKING TIME: 15 MINUTES • **SERVES 4**

12	ounces penne or ziti pasta
1	pound sugar snap peas, strings removed
1/3	cup snipped fresh dill
3	scallions, thinly sliced
3/4	cup chicken broth
3	tablespoons reduced-fat sour cream
1	tablespoon unsalted butter
1	teaspoon grated lemon zest
2	tablespoons lemon juice
1/2	teaspoon salt
4	ounces smoked salmon, slivered

1. In large pot of boiling water, cook pasta according to package directions until firm-tender. Add sugar snaps to water during final 1 minute of cooking; drain.

2. Meanwhile, in a large bowl, combine dill, scallions, broth, sour cream, butter, lemon zest, lemon juice, and salt. Add hot pasta and sugar snaps, tossing well. Add smoked salmon and toss again.

Calories: 450, fat: 7 g, saturated fat: 4 g, sodium: 850 mg, carbohydrate: 75 g, protein: 21 g.

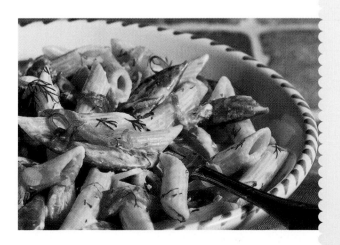

Creole-Style Beans

Robust beans, a prime source for folate, are cooked with the traditional Creole trinity of celery, onion, and green pepper, which offer up vitamins C, B₆, and more folate. The tomatoes give the dish vitamins C and E.

PREPARATION TIME: 10 MINUTES, PLUS OVERNIGHT SOAKING
COOKING TIME: 1 HOUR 15 MINUTES • **SERVES 4**

3/4	cup dried cannellini or navy beans
1	teaspoon olive oil
3/4	cup vegetable broth
1	small fresh red chile, seeded and finely chopped (you may want to substitute 1/4-1/2 teaspoon red pepper flakes)
1	garlic clove, minced
3	celery stalks, chopped
1/3	cup chopped onion
1	green bell pepper, seeded and chopped
1	teaspoon paprika
1	bay leaf
1	can (14 ounces) diced tomatoes

1. In a medium bowl, combine beans and enough water to cover by 2 inches, and let soak, chilled in refrigerator, overnight.

2. Drain beans in a colander, and rinse well under cold water. In large saucepan, combine beans with enough water to cover. Boil rapidly for 15 minutes, skimming surface as necessary. Drain and rinse well and set aside.

3. Add oil, 1 tablespoon broth, pepper flakes, garlic, celery, onion, and green pepper to saucepan. Cook mixture, covered, over medium heat, shaking pan occasionally until vegetables have softened, about 10 minutes. Stir in paprika and cook, stirring, for 1 minute. Add bay leaf, boiled beans, remaining broth and tomatoes and simmer, covered, until beans are tender, about 45 minutes, removing lid for last 10 minutes so that juices reduce. Season with salt and pepper to taste.

Calories: 100, fat: 2 g, saturated fat: 0 g, sodium: 125 mg, carbohydrate: 18 g, protein: 5 g.

Risotto with Spring Vegetables

This wholesome risotto is packed with fresh vegetables, which offer vitamins B6, C, E, and folate from the asparagus, vitamin C and folate from the beans, vitamin C and calcium from the peas, vitamin C and folate from the leek, not to mention even more calcium from the cheese.

PREPARATION TIME: 20 MINUTES, PLUS 5 MINUTES STANDING
COOKING TIME: 40–45 MINUTES • **SERVES 4**

4	cups vegetable broth
1/4	teaspoon crumbled saffron threads
2	tablespoons olive oil
3	carrots, chopped
2	garlic cloves, crushed
1/2	cup chopped well-washed leek
1/2	pound Arborio rice
1/4	pound (about 8) asparagus spears, cut into 1-inch lengths
1/4	pound green beans, cut into 1-inch lengths
3/4	cup green peas, defrosted if frozen
1/4	cup chopped fresh herbs, such as chives, dill, flat-leaved parsley and tarragon
1/2	cup grated Parmesan cheese

1. In a saucepan, warm broth, then add saffron and let stand off heat for 10 minutes.

2. Meanwhile, in a large skillet heat oil over medium-low heat, add carrots, garlic, and leek and cook, stirring, until softened, about 10 minutes. Add rice to vegetables and stir for 1 minute or until grains are glossy.

3. Return broth to heat and keep at a simmer. Add a ladleful of broth to the rice, stirring continuously until it has been absorbed. Continue adding broth, a ladleful at a time, and stirring for 15 minutes.

4. Add asparagus, beans, and peas to rice and continue stirring and adding stock until rice and vegetables are tender. (This should take 15–20 minutes). Remove pan from heat, stir in herbs and Parmesan, and let rest, covered, for 5 minutes. Season with salt and pepper to taste.

Calories: 390, fat: 13 g, saturated fat: 4 g, sodium: 240 mg, carbohydrate: 58 g, protein: 15 g.

Tex-Mex Turkey, Corn, & Barley Casserole

Barley gives you vitamin B6 and folate, among other good things. You get even more B6 from the turkey and peppers in this hearty dish.

PREPARATION TIME: 10–12 MINUTES **COOKING TIME:** 1 HOUR 15 MINUTES • **SERVES 4**

- 2 tablespoons canola oil
- 2 onions, coarsely chopped
- 1 large red or green bell pepper, coarsely chopped
- 1 teaspoon finely chopped hot chile pepper
- 1 cup pearl barley, sorted and rinsed
- 1 3/4 cups chicken broth
- 1 can (14 ounces) crushed tomatoes
- 1/8 teaspoon each salt and pepper
- 2 cups shredded cooked turkey
- 1 cup frozen corn kernels, thawed

1. Preheat oven to 325°F. In a flameproof casserole, heat oil over moderate heat. Sauté onions, bell pepper, and chile pepper, stirring, about 7 minutes or until softened and lightly browned.

2. Add barley and cook, stirring, until well coated with oil. Pour in chicken broth and crushed tomatoes, and season with salt and pepper.

3. Bring to a boil, then stir in turkey. Cover casserole and cook in oven, stirring occasionally, about 55 minutes or until almost all liquid has been absorbed and barley is nearly tender.

4. Stir in corn kernels, cover casserole, and cook 5 to 10 minutes longer, until heated through.

Calories: 475, fat: 9 g, saturated fat: 2 g, sodium: 262 mg, carbohydrate: 65 g, protein: 31 g.

Herbed Polenta

The milk and cheese in this recipe give you calcium; the cornmeal provides some vitamin B6.

PREPARATION TIME: 5 MINUTES PLUS CHILLING TIME **COOKING TIME:** 25 MINUTES • **SERVES 6**

- 1 cup yellow cornmeal
- 2 cups 1% low-fat milk
- 1/8 teaspoon each salt and pepper
- 2 tablespoons chopped parsley or basil
- 2 tablespoons finely grated Parmesan cheese

1. Combine cornmeal with 1 cup water in small bowl. In nonstick saucepan, bring milk and 1 cup water to a boil. Season with salt and pepper.

2. Reduce heat slightly and slowly stir cornmeal into milk mixture. Cook, stirring constantly, about 5 minutes or until mixture boils and thickens slightly.

3. Reduce heat to very low and simmer polenta gently, stirring frequently, about 10 minutes or until the mixture is smooth and thickened.

4. Remove saucepan from heat. Add chopped herbs and cheese and stir well to mix thoroughly.

5. Turn polenta out onto a nonstick baking pan and spread to a depth of 1/4 inch with a palette knife. Chill for 2 hours to set. Preheat broiler.

6. With a cookie cutter, cut rounds from polenta. Use trimmings to make more. Or cut into 6 wedges. Broil on a rack about 5 minutes, until golden.

Calories: 128, fat: 2 g, saturated fat: 1 g, sodium: 128 mg, carbohydrate: 22 g, protein: 6 g.

Apricot-Maple Acorn Squash

Acorn squash, with its bright orange flesh, gives you lots of vitamin C and vitamin B$_6$. With maple syrup and apricot jam, it's delectable.

COOKING TIME: 1 HOUR OR UNTIL TENDER • **SERVES 4**

- 2 one-pound acorn squashes
- 1/4 cup apricot jam
- 2 tablespoons maple syrup

1. Halve and seed the squashes.

2. Place in baking pan, cut sides down, add 1/3 cup water, cover with foil, and bake for 25 minutes at 400°F. Drain. Turn cut sides up.

3. Stir together apricot jam and maple syrup. Spoon into squash. Bake 35 minutes or until tender.

Calories: 170, fat: 0 g, saturated fat: 0 g, sodium: 15 mg, carbohydrate: 43 g, protein: 2 g.

Orange-Glazed Carrots

This is a way to make your vitamin C— from carrots and oranges—irresistible.

PREPARATION TIME: 5 MINUTES
COOKING TIME: 15 MINUTES • **SERVES 4**

- 1 pound very small, peeled carrots (or pre-peeled "baby" carrots)
- 1/4 cup orange juice
- 2 tablespoons orange marmalade (or apricot jam)
- 2 teaspoons unsalted butter
- 1/2 teaspoon salt

1. In a saucepan with a steamer insert, cook carrots over water until crisp-tender.

2. In a large skillet, heat orange juice, marmalade (or apricot jam), butter, and salt.

3. Add carrots and cook over moderate heat until nicely glazed.

Calories: 90, fat: 3 g, saturated fat: 2 g, sodium: 280 mg, carbohydrate: 17 g, protein: 1 g.

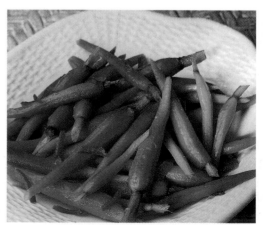
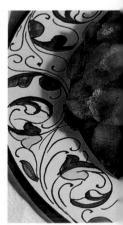

Potato Torte

For people with arthritis, potatoes' great assets are vitamins B$_6$ and C. In this recipe Parmesan cheese gives you an added shot of calcium.

PREPARATION TIME: 10 MINUTES
COOKING TIME: 50 MINUTES • **SERVES 4**

- 5 teaspoons olive oil
- 2 pounds baking potatoes, peeled and very thinly sliced
- 3/4 teaspoon each salt and pepper
- 1/4 cup grated Parmesan cheese
- 2 scallions, thinly sliced
- 3 tablespoons snipped fresh dill

1. Preheat oven to 450°F. Brush a 9-inch pie plate with 1 teaspoon oil. Cover bottom with an overlapping layer of potatoes, using one-fourth of total. Sprinkle with 1 teaspoon oil, 1/4 teaspoon each salt and pepper, 1 tablespoon Parmesan, one-third of scallions, and 1 tablespoon dill.

2. Repeat for 2 more layers. Top with final layer of potatoes, 1 teaspoon oil, and 1 tablespoon Parmesan. Place an empty pie plate or round baking dish on top of potatoes and bake in lower third of oven for 50 minutes or until potatoes are crusty on bottom (lift gently with a spatula to check) and tender throughout.

3. Cool in pan for 5 minutes before loosening bottom and sides with a small spatula and inverting onto a platter.

Calories: 290, fat: 8 g, saturated fat: 2 g, sodium: 500 mg, carbohydrate: 49 g, protein: 9 g.

Sweet Potato & Apple Bake

Unlike the familiar marshmallow topping, apples make a substantial nutritional contribution to a sweet-potato casserole, which abounds in vitamin C from the sweet potatoes, apples, onion, and lemon juice plus B$_6$ from the sweet potatoes.

PREPARATION TIME: 20 MINUTES, **COOKING TIME:** 45 MINUTES • **SERVES 4**

- 1 tablespoon unsalted butter
- 1 onion, finely chopped
- 2 pounds sweet potatoes, peeled and thinly sliced
- 2 McIntosh apples, cut into 1/2-inch-thick wedges
- 3 tablespoons sugar
- 2 tablespoons lemon juice
- 3/4 cup chicken broth
- 1/2 teaspoon salt
- 1/4 teaspoon pepper

1. Preheat oven to 450°F. In a very large nonstick skillet, heat butter over moderate heat. Add onion and sauté for 5 minutes or until tender.

2. Add sweet potatoes, apples, 2 tablespoons sugar, and lemon juice, and cook until sugar has melted. Add broth, salt, and pepper, and bring to a boil.

3. Transfer mixture to a 7 x 11-inch glass baking dish. Cover with foil and bake for 25 minutes or until sweet potatoes are tender. Uncover, sprinkle with remaining 1 tablespoon sugar, and bake for 10 minutes or until lightly browned.

Calories: 350, fat: 4 g, saturated fat: 2 g, sodium: 290 mg, carbohydrate: 76 g, protein: 5 g.

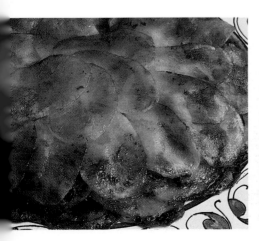

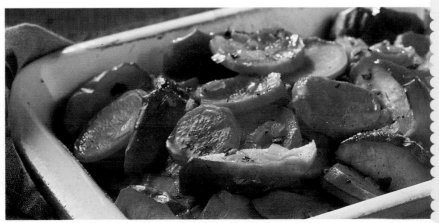

Roasted New Potatoes

New potatoes, full of vitamins C and B₆, appear in the late spring or early summer. Enjoy!

PREPARATION TIME: 10 MINUTES,
COOKING TIME: 45 MINUTES • **SERVES 8**

1 1/2	pounds small new potatoes, scrubbed
3	cloves garlic, thinly sliced
2	tablespoons olive or canola oil
1/2	teaspoon crumbled rosemary (optional)

1. Preheat oven to 400°F. In a large bowl, combine potatoes with garlic, oil, and rosemary, if using.

2. Transfer to a roasting pan, arranging in one layer, and roast about 45 minutes or until golden and cooked through.

Calories: 219, fat: 8 g, saturated fat: 1 g, sodium: 16 mg, carbohydrate: 35 g, protein: 3 g.

Sweet Roasted Squash with Shallots

Roasted vegetables are sweetened with a touch of maple syrup. It's a lovely way to get your vitamin C and folate from both the shallots and the squash.

PREPARATION TIME: 15 MINUTES
COOKING TIME: 30–35 MINUTES • **SERVES 4**

2	pounds butternut squash
8	shallots, peeled
3	sprigs fresh thyme
1	teaspoon olive oil
2	teaspoons pure maple syrup, or light honey

1. Preheat oven to 375°F. Halve squash lengthwise, scrape out seeds, and remove peel with a vegetable peeler. Cut into 1 1/4-inch cubes.

2. Combine squash, shallots, thyme, oil, syrup, and salt and pepper to taste in a roasting pan and toss to coat vegetables. Roast vegetables until they are tender and golden brown, 30–35 minutes, turning occasionally.

Calories: 120, fat: 2 g, saturated fat: 0 g, sodium: 10 mg, carbohydrate: 29 g, protein: 2 g.

Caramelized Orange Compote

Oranges are a prime source of vitamin C; here's a way to dress them up.

PREPARATION TIME: 10 MINUTES
COOKING TIME: 2 MINUTES • **SERVES 4**

- 4 peeled and segmented navel oranges
- 1/4 cup brown sugar
- 1/4 teaspoon cinnamon
- 1 tablespoon slivered orange zest

1. Preheat broiler. Place peeled and segmented navel oranges in gratin dish or shallow broilerproof baking dish.

2. Sprinkle with brown sugar, cinnamon, and zest. Broil 2 minutes or until sugar melts.

Calories: 120, fat: 0 g, saturated fat: 0 g, sodium: 5 mg, carbohydrate: 30 g, protein: 1 g.

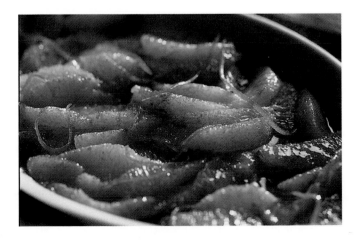

Chocolate-Hazelnut Cheesecake

Toasted hazelnuts top this velvety tofu and cottage cheese (major sources of calcium) cheesecake. The egg offers vitamin D; the canola oil, omega-3 fatty acids.

PREPARATION TIME: 15 MINUTES
COOKING TIME: 50 MINUTES
CHILLING TIME: 2 HOURS • **SERVES 12**

- 1/3 cup hazelnuts
- 1 cup graham cracker crumbs (5 ounces)
- 1 tablespoon canola oil
- 1/4 cup unsweetened cocoa powder
- 1 pound silken tofu
- 1 cup creamed (4%) cottage cheese
- 1 ounce semisweet chocolate, melted
- 1/2 cup granulated sugar
- 2/3 cup packed light brown sugar
- 2 tablespoons flour
- 1 egg
- 2 egg whites
- 1 teaspoon vanilla extract

1. Preheat oven to 375°F. Toast hazelnuts on a baking sheet for 7 minutes or until skins begin to crinkle. (Leave the oven on.) Transfer hazelnuts to a kitchen towel and rub to remove as much of the skin as possible (some skin will remain). When hazelnuts are cool enough to handle, coarsely chop and set aside.

2. In a small bowl, stir together crumbs, oil, and 1 tablespoon water. Press mixture into bottom and partway up sides of a 9 1/2-inch springform pan. Bake for 8 minutes or until crust is set. Cool on a rack. Reduce oven temperature to 350°F.

3. In a small bowl, combine cocoa and 1/4 cup water until well moistened. In a food processor, combine tofu, cottage cheese, melted semisweet chocolate, granulated sugar, brown sugar, flour, whole egg, egg whites, vanilla, and cocoa mixture, and process until very smooth.

4. Pour batter into prepared crust and bake for 40 minutes. Reduce oven temperature to 250°F, sprinkle nuts on top, and bake for 10 minutes or until cheesecake is just set. Cool to room temperature; refrigerate for 2 hours or until chilled.

Calories: 210, fat: 7 g, saturated fat: 2 g, sodium: 190 mg, carbohydrate: 30 g, protein: 8 g.

Berry Sorbet

Sorbets, made only from fruit and sweetener—no milk—are fat and cholesterol free. You'll always have room for a dessert as light and refreshing as this one, particularly when it is packed with vitamin C from lime juice and both kinds of berries.

PREPARATION TIME: 8 MINUTES
COOKING TIME: 3 MINUTES
FREEZING TIME: 5 HOURS • **MAKES SIX 1/2-CUP SERVINGS.**

- 1/2 cup lime juice
- 2 tablespoons grenadine syrup or 2 tablespoons water plus 1 tablespoon sugar
- 1/3 cup water
- 1 package (12 ounces) frozen unsweetened raspberries, thawed
- 1 package (12 ounces) frozen unsweetened strawberries, thawed

1. In a medium saucepan, bring lime juice, sugar, grenadine, and water to a boil over moderate heat. Cook about 1 minute or until sugar is dissolved.

2. In a food processor or blender, whirl raspberries and strawberries for 30 seconds or until pureed. Press fruit through a fine sieve to eliminate seeds. You should have 2 cups of puree; if not, add enough water to make 2 cups.

3. Stir puree into sugar syrup until well combined. Transfer mixture to an 8" x 8" x 2" pan, cover with plastic wrap, and freeze for 2 hours or until the center is almost frozen. Remove sorbet from freezer and beat until smooth. Return to freezer for 45 minutes, then beat again until smooth. Freeze 2 to 3 hours more before serving.

Calories: 125, fat: 0 g, saturated fat: 0 g, sodium: 1 mg, carbohydrate: 33 g, protein: 1 g.

Pineapple Foster

Bananas Foster is a beloved New Orleans dessert, created in the 1950s at Brennan's Restaurant. This pineapple variation, in which the fruit is a good source of vitamin C, will bring raves. The frozen yogurt adds calcium as well as a cool taste contrast.

PREPARATION TIME: 15 MINUTES
COOKING TIME: 10 MINUTES • **SERVES 4**

- 4 teaspoons unsalted butter
- 3 tablespoons packed light brown sugar
- 1/4 teaspoon ground nutmeg
- 6 slices (3/4 inch thick) fresh pineapple, cored and cut into quarters
- 3 tablespoons dark rum
- 2 tablespoons Grand Marnier, or other orange liqueur
- 1 1/3 cups vanilla frozen yogurt

1. In a large skillet, melt butter over moderate heat. When it begins to foam, add brown sugar and nutmeg, and heat until sugar has melted. Add pineapple and cook, tossing often, for 4 minutes or until pineapple is warmed through.

2. Remove pan from heat, sprinkle rum and Grand Marnier over pineapple, and ignite alcohol with a long match. Return pan to heat and shake until alcohol burns off.

3. Serve the pineapple slices and sauce with the frozen yogurt.

Calories: 280, fat: 5 g, saturated fat: 3 g, sodium: 35 mg, carbohydrate: 48 g, protein: 5 g.

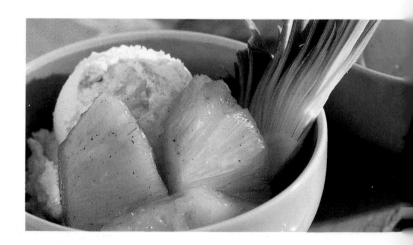

Boldface page references indicate exercise instructions.

About the Authors

Richard Laliberte is a veteran health journalist whose articles have appeared in *Glamour, Redbook, Woman's Day, Ladies' Home Journal, Fitness, Shape, Men's Journal, Self*, and many other magazines. He also has been a contributing editor at *Cooking Light* and *Parents* magazines, and was a senior editor and writer at *Men's Health*. He has written several books on health and fitness, including *Stopping Diabetes in Its Tracks* and *The Doctor's Guide to Chronic Pain*. He lives in eastern Pennsylvania with his wife and two children.

Virginia B. Kraus, M.D., Ph.D., is a rheumatologist and an associate professor of medicine, Division of Rheumatology, at the Center for Human Genetics at Duke University Medical Center. She is the principal investigator at Duke University for a major effort to identify the genes responsible for hereditary forms of osteoarthritis. Dr. Kraus also investigates markers of arthritis measured in body fluids. This research could lead to more effective monitoring of the disease's progression in the human body. She is a member of a multidisciplinary team at Duke recently awarded a large grant from the Arthritis Institute of the National Institutes of Health to study the role of inflammation in osteoarthritis and the impact of a comprehensive therapeutic strategy of weight loss, exercise, and pain management for knee osteoarthritis.

Daniel S. Rooks, Ph.D., is the director of the Be Well! Tanger Center for Health Management and an investigator in the Division of Rheumatology at Beth Israel Deaconess Medical Center in Boston. He is also an assistant professor of medicine at Harvard Medical School. Dr. Rooks's research centers on chronic disease self-management. His current work examines exercise, nutrition, education, and behavioral interventions in people with osteoarthritis, fibromyalgia, and obesity. He received a doctor of science degree in applied anatomy and physiology from Boston University, and is a current recipient of an Arthritis Investigator Award from the Arthritis Foundation.